FERTILITY
TECHNOLOGY

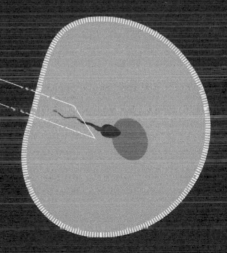

The MIT Press Essential Knowledge Series

A complete list of books in this series can be found online at
https://mitpress.mit.edu/books/series/mit-press-essential-knowledge-series.

FERTILITY TECHNOLOGY

DONNA J. DRUCKER

The MIT Press | Cambridge, Massachusetts | London, England

The MIT Press would like to thank the anonymous peer reviewers who provided comments on drafts of this book. The generous work of academic experts is essential for establishing the authority and quality of our publications. We acknowledge with gratitude the contributions of these otherwise uncredited readers.

This book was set in Chaparral Pro by New Best-set Typesetters Ltd. Printed and bound in the United States of America.

Library of Congress Cataloging-in-Publication Data

Names: Drucker, Donna J., author.
Title: Fertility technology / Donna J. Drucker.
Description: Cambridge, Massachusetts : The MIT Press, [2023] | Series: The MIT Press essential knowledge series | Includes bibliographical references and index.
Identifiers: LCCN 2022011344 (print) | LCCN 2022011345 (ebook) | ISBN 9780262544696 (paperback) | ISBN 9780262372329 (epub) | ISBN 9780262372336 (pdf)
Subjects: LCSH: Human reproductive technology. | Fertility.
Classification: LCC RG133.5 .D78 2023 (print) | LCC RG133.5 (ebook) | DDC 618.1/7806—dc23/eng/20220629
LC record available at https://lccn.loc.gov/2022011344
LC ebook record available at https://lccn.loc.gov/2022011345

10 9 8 7 6 5 4 3 2 1

CONTENTS

SERIES FOREWORD

The MIT Press Essential Knowledge series offers accessible, concise, beautifully produced pocket-size books on topics of current interest. Written by leading thinkers, the books in this series deliver expert overviews of subjects that range from the cultural and the historical to the scientific and the technical.

In today's era of instant information gratification, we have ready access to opinions, rationalizations, and superficial descriptions. Much harder to come by is the foundational knowledge that informs a principled understanding of the world. Essential Knowledge books fill that need. Synthesizing specialized subject matter for nonspecialists and engaging critical topics through fundamentals, each of these compact volumes offers readers a point of access to complex ideas.

PREFACE

This book, like others in the field of reproductive studies, must balance the relevance of "women" and "men" as categories of personhood with specific historical meaning and the necessary inclusion of transgender and non-binary individuals, whose ability to become pregnant or to impregnate someone else may not correlate to their gender identity. I use gendered terms when needed to discuss particular experiences of self-identified women and men in the past and use gender-neutral terms as much as possible.

This book is not a guide to choosing a fertility method. Please consult a health care practitioner for advice.

TECHNOLOGY FOR FERTILITY

In the late 1850s, a twenty-eight-year-old woman approached the Woman's Hospital in New York City. She had been married for nine years and "was willing to try anything" to conceive a child.[1] One of the physicians there used a syringe and glass tube to inject half a drop of her husband's sperm into her uterus. On the tenth try, she conceived and carried the fetus for four months until miscarrying. The woman's name is lost to history, though her experience was recorded in the work of Dr. J. Marion Sims (1813–1883), a renowned American gynecologist. Sims's treatment of this woman was the first time that a physician admitted publicly to trying artificial insemination (what he termed "artificial fertilization") with medical technology.[2] Though Sims was unsuccessful—this was the only pregnancy out of his fifty-five attempts at using the syringe-tube combination, and it did not result in a live birth—his description of using medical tools for artificial insemination inspired other medical professionals to try using technologies to assist patients with their quest for a child.

This book is a history and analysis of the following principal types of fertility technologies from the 1860s to the present: (1) devices and techniques related to artificial insemination (AI); (2) diagnostic tools and surgical techniques, particularly insufflation and salpingogram apparatuses; (3) ovulation timing in a monthly cycle; (4) in vitro fertilization (IVF) and its associated and subsequent developments; and (5) sperm, egg, and embryo freezing. This book is organized chronologically according to the first recorded use of each technology, and then traces the offshoots of the original technology into the present. It focuses on each technology's development, dispersion, and use in humans but includes use for animals where relevant. It argues that fertility technologies are not neutral—their innovation and use have both reflected and shaped how people think about reproduction, family, race, and kinship from the mid-nineteenth century through the present. As Katharine Dow writes, "How we reproduce seems to say something about who we are and who we want to be and because of a sense that future generations are the product of parents' reproductive decision-making."[3]

It is important to note that the study of fertility technology and the study of fertility and infertility are not the

Fertility technologies
are not neutral.

same. The World Health Organization (WHO), for example, uses a medical definition of infertility: "infertility is a disease of the male or female reproductive system defined by the failure to achieve a pregnancy after twelve months or more of regular unprotected sexual intercourse." Depending on the context and situation, infertility can be a disease, a story, a disorder, a chronic illness, a form of suffering, a disability—or some combination of the above.[4] It eludes a singular definition.

There are many nuances in sociocultural understandings of infertility that are harder to find in the historical record. For example, records may not distinguish between primary infertility (no live births) and secondary infertility (aka subfertility, not more than one birth without assisted reproductive technologies [ARTs]). Women not seeking pregnancy may be infertile without knowing it—or it not mattering to them. Records created by elites, however (and especially elites in the medical profession), privilege the construction of fertility or infertility as a medical condition.[5] If infertility is categorizable as a medical condition, then it follows that it has (or could have) a medical treatment, and many physicians followed this line of thinking as they sought technological and surgical cures for their patients. This book traces advances and experiments in medical practice, which often take place in the most industrialized countries. It also provides a broader picture of the reception of these technologies around the

The study of fertility
technology and the
study of fertility
and infertility are not
the same.

world, and of how child-seekers used technologies on their own terms to try and manifest pregnancies, births, and families according to their own vision.

This chapter introduces the following chapters and the key concepts of the book, and it considers why people seek a "technological fix" for fertility problems in the first place.[6] It is no coincidence that physicians and patients started to look for technological assistance in the mid-nineteenth century, when industrial capitalism and colonialism were at worldwide peaks of influence. The world was awash in new technologies, to put it mildly, and the absence of wanted pregnancy was yet another medical problem that could potentially be solved with the application of appropriate technology.

The second chapter traces the development of six different technologies in use from the mid-nineteenth century to the mid-twentieth century. Beginning in the mid-nineteenth century, gynecologists used the relatively simple combination of a cannula and syringe to place fresh semen as deep as they could into the vagina—and past the cervix into the uterus if possible. In the 1910s and 1920s, physicians using this technique added a stem pessary or cervical cap to the process after the seminal injection to hold the fluid in place. Likewise in this era, physicians sometimes prescribed hormonal supplements, and they began to use insufflation apparatuses or salpingograms to check for and to remove blockages in the fallopian tubes, sometimes followed with AI. However, the ideal timing for the injection of semen was guesswork until Dr. Kyusaku Ogino (1882–1975) and Dr. Hermann H. Knaus (1892–1970) confirmed the timing of ovulation in a woman's monthly cycle. Once the timing of egg maturation could (roughly) be established, ovulation timing trackers could be either combined with insufflation and AI or used on their own, particularly for married Roman Catholic couples.

The timing of ovulation also provided the medical groundwork for the focus of the third chapter, which describes the discovery of IVF, its successor technologies, and its infrastructures. It describes the work of those who made significant advances in innovation and development, including Dr. Patrick Steptoe (1913–1988), Dr. Robert Edwards (1925–2013), and Jean Purdy (1945–1985), who were the first scientists to fertilize an ovum outside the uterus that resulted in a live birth. It traces how scientists and physicians attempted to improve the accuracy of IVF through techniques such as gamete intrafallopian transfer (GIFT) and zygote intrafallopian transfer (ZIFT) in the 1980s, the pathbreaking advance of intracytoplasmic sperm injection (ICSI) in the early 1990s, and those used to examine embryos before implantation, including preimplantation genetic diagnosis (PGD) and preimplantation genetic testing for aneuploidy (PGT-A, known previously as preimplantation genetic screening [PGS]).

Additionally, laboratories, surgical rooms, transport systems, and tissue banks with all of their intersecting technologies are parts of the infrastructures that make the use of these techniques possible.

The fourth chapter identifies the advantages and problems of using these technologies in different legal, ethical, and religious contexts and how fertility travel has become commonplace. Identifying such differences shows how geographic location, political histories, and religious belief systems can structure the ways that people do and do not use fertility technologies and services and the aftereffects of their use in families and communities. The presence of these technologies in the global medical landscape raises the fundamental ethical and moral question of who state and medical authorities allow to use them—and how making access illegal to some persons points them toward low-tech instead of high-tech means of assisted reproduction, or to seeking services or tissues available in other countries. It is clear that "reproductive ethics are not only about individuals' or couples' private decisions about whether and how to have children but also about what is socially, morally, and legally acceptable to the larger community."[7]

Furthermore, restrictions on fertility technology use on account of age, sexual orientation, religious prohibition, or a desire for privacy lead many child-seekers to fertility travel. Such travel includes accessing services with fewer restrictions on patients (higher age limits for intended mothers, for example), importing provider gametes from abroad for cost or genetic reasons (including resemblance to the intended parent[s]), paying for the providers to travel to the intended mother or surrogate, and hiring an overseas surrogate to gestate a child with one's own or donor gametes. Legal restrictions, cold-chain technologies, and fertility clinics' profit interests structure the worldwide movement of people and gametes, creating what some scholars call "fertility travel," "reproflows," and "reproscapes"—the movement of people and genetic material from one country to another. Indeed, "people accessing treatments are part of a global reproductive ecology, in which actions affecting their life experiences can occur far away from them."[8]

The fifth chapter considers how technologies affect ideals and realities of kinship and family. It examines the ways that race became a key part of AI and ARTs generally, first as part of sperm-donor catalogs in the early 1980s and later as part of individual efforts to manufacture kinship through physical resemblance and "whitening" one's offspring. It then turns to feminist critique of ARTs and the role that reproductive justice plays in identifying which legal efforts support individual autonomy over reproductive choices and healthy children's futures. It concludes with a reflection on the financial and personal costs of ARTs on child-seekers and considers their criteria for deciding to continue their efforts or not.

The sixth chapter identifies current research on fertility technologies and future directions in their innovation. It provides insight into the expanding for-profit fertility industry and its promotion of add-ons. It outlines the growing research on pregnancy and the use of fertility technologies among non-binary and trans individuals and points toward the higher need for specialized reproductive health care services. Further, research on uterine transplants from both living and deceased donors suggests a future in which patients could gestate and bring a pregnancy to term if they were assigned male at birth (AMAB), and in which the gender assignment of any parent at birth does not factor into reproduction at all.

There are four key concepts threading through this book. The first is the legal status of fertility technology in different countries over time, including which technologies are legal or illegal for all, who can or cannot use them, whether gametes can be removed from the country and transported elsewhere and whether a country's fertility clinics and citizens can import gametes, and whether the state supports fertility, especially in the form of covering IVF treatments through public health insurance. A second key concept is the role of fertility technology in the history of women, gender, and sexuality, and particularly its role in wider struggles for legal and political rights, autonomy, and reproductive justice. Though feminist writers in the 1980s castigated ARTs as part of patriarchal control of women's bodies, feminists have more recently directed their attention to equality of access to ARTs and to patterns of abuse and neglect of surrogates and egg donors.

A third key concept is that advances in fertility technology take place along two paths: the development of diagnostic tools (such as tubal insufflation to determine blocked fallopian tubes) and the development of treatment mechanisms, most prominently ARTs. Both types of technologies are necessary for helping individuals and couples to achieve pregnancy, though neither of them cures infertility. A fourth key concept is that identical technologies can be used to promote fertility and for contraception. For example, cervical caps can be used either to keep sperm inside the uterus after an AI treatment or during heterosexual intercourse to keep sperm out.[9] The same is true for ovulation tracking via cervical mucus, cervical shape, and basal body temperature (BBT). Together, these four key concepts show that technologies have been deeply interwoven with attempts to achieve pregnancy for over a century and a half and that low-tech and high-tech methods are in use unequally across the world. The most technically advanced methods are developed, tested, and used in countries with the most sophisticated medical infrastructures, and these advancements happen so quickly that regulatory agencies and medical researchers have a hard time staying up-to-date. This situation leads to for-profit fertility companies promoting pricey unregulated or untested add-ons, which may do nothing at best and may cause harm at worst.

Comparing global patterns of technological innovation, adoption, access, regulation, and use illustrates how fertility technologies can both benefit people who want children and exacerbate inequality and health problems for those who provide gametes or other bodily services, particularly as egg donors and surrogates. Such comparisons also highlight the roles of hospital and laboratory infrastructure, health insurance, and well-trained medical professionals in making the healthy and safe use of high-tech fertility technologies possible. But increasingly specialized, expensive, and high-tech methods are not the only way forward. On account of accessibility, cost, health, or other reasons, many people use low-tech fertility methods, such as the low-cost IVF methods developed by the Walking Egg Project in Ghana and home-use kits adapted from Sims's original model.

This book's focus on fertility technology illustrates the ongoing difficulty of achieving pregnancy in the face of anatomical, physiological, or genetic obstacles. A focus in popular media on extreme cases, such as more than six fetuses carried to term by one mother, or healthy pregnancies and live deliveries by women in their fifties or early sixties, fosters expectations for fertility technologies that they cannot meet for everyone.[10] It also makes clear that diagnosing fertility problems is a different matter than achieving pregnancy or curing infertility. And despite advances in fertility technology, especially over the past two decades, "hope technology" can still take many child-seekers only so far.[11]

FERTILITY TECHNOLOGY BEFORE IVF

This chapter provides a historical overview of fertility technologies that were in use before IVF, some of which are still used in the present. The technologies examined below—syringes and cannulas, stem pessaries, hormone supplements, pelvic surgeries, insufflation apparatuses and salpingograms, ovulation timing, and sperm banks—show that technologies for fertility developed unevenly across the world from the 1860s onward.[1] Some required medical supervision, and others did not; some were painful, and others were not. Examining them gives insight into the various ways that physicians, manufacturers, entrepreneurs, and patients all looked to technology as a possible means to diagnose, treat, and overcome medical problems in order to achieve pregnancy.

Records of artificial insemination attempts with animals date back centuries.

Artificial Insemination

Records of artificial insemination attempts with animals date back centuries, most famously to Lazzaro Spallanzani (1729–1799) and his experiments on dogs.[2] There are different years in which a technological history of fertility assistance in humans could begin, as scattered references to artificial insemination efforts were occasionally recorded. In the late eighteenth century, an English draper and his wife were having trouble conceiving, and a physician called John Hunter helped them. Hunter advised them to first have intercourse (ensuring that the wife was stimulated enough to have the orgasm he and others still considered essential to conception) and then to have ready a warm syringe "fitted for the purpose" to collect and then inject his semen into his wife's vagina. It is unclear if this event actually occurred, as "dates of occurrence range from 1776–1799 and the specifics range from Hunter providing the husband with a syringe to Hunter performing it himself," but the story of Hunter's (and the couple's) success became part of the historical record.[3] In 1869, the French physician Louis Girault reported that following operations on forty previously sterile women beginning in 1838, eighteen of them bore children. He supposedly blew semen into patients' vaginas through a hollow cannula two days after menstruation ceased, gathering semen by "'la méthode Française' (masturbation) or 'la méthode

Américaine' (syringed from the vaginal basin immediately after intercourse)."[4] However, this history starts with J. Marion Sims's documentation of his attempt at artificial insemination using a syringe and cannula in *Clinical Notes on Uterine Surgery* (1866), as it had a distinct technological and practice-based impact on US and European gynecology.

Sims based his gynecological research on enslaved women in the Slave Hospital in Montgomery, Alabama, from 1845 to 1849 and on free women at the Woman's Hospital in New York City starting in 1855. As Deirdre Cooper Owens writes, "Sims depended on enslaved black women's bodies to discover cures for vesico-vaginal fistulae and [to] perfect surgical instruments such as the duck-billed speculum, achievements that were responsible for his global status as a pioneering gynecological surgeon."[5] The artificial insemination experiment that he outlined in *Clinical Notes on Uterine Surgery* was notable not for its success—as mentioned in chapter 1, only one out of fifty-five patients achieved pregnancy, and she miscarried after four months—but for the description of the syringe and cannula that Sims used to assist with that pregnancy. Two images of the tools that he used appeared next to his description, visually reinforcing his point that the tools themselves were simple and replicable by readers. The description likewise indicated compassion for infertile women (a feeling certainly not extended to his enslaved patients, who could not give consent). As Margaret Marsh and Wanda Ronner observe, "His ideas seemed to 'work,' perhaps not in the sense that he made the sterile fertile . . . but that he convinced his patients that his instruments and his surgical expertise provided them with more hope of relief—from their pelvic pain, their dysmenorrhea, and their sterility—than any dietary prescriptions, gradual instrumental therapy, or self-help could do."[6]

By the 1860s, even though Sims had been dismissed from the Woman's Hospital for permitting non-physicians to watch operations in its surgical theater, he had become one of the best-known and widely read gynecologists in the United States and Europe.[7] The fact that his books, articles, and autobiography were translated and republished helped manifest the 1860s and 1870s as watershed decades in medical developments surrounding pregnancy and birth, including the establishment of embryology as an academic field, the increased visibility of fetuses in medical schools and textbooks, women giving birth in hospitals under male medical supervision instead of at home, and the growing number of state laws against abortion.[8] As *Clinical Notes on Uterine Surgery* was translated into German and French the same year that it was published in English in the United States and England, physicians who read any of these languages could understand Sims's description of AI and could begin to experiment with the technique themselves.[9]

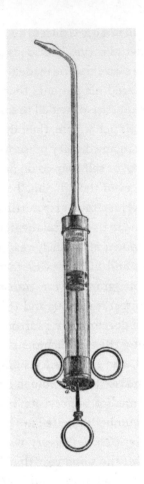

Figure 1 Syringe for artificial insemination depicted in J. Marion Sims, *Clinical Notes on Uterine Surgery* (1866). *Source:* Courtesy National Library of Medicine, Bethesda, Maryland.

Additionally, in other publications, he outlined his process for examining postcoital sperm under a microscope to look for abnormalities, drawing attention to the fact that infertility was not only a female problem; spermatic health could likewise play a role. Another US physician, Max Huhner (1873–1947), advanced Sims's examination practices and designed a test to determine postcoital sperm motility microscopically. The correlation of the Sims-Huhner test (or postcoital test [PCT]) with the chance of pregnancy has been debated among gynecologists ever since Huhner first published his method in 1913.[10]

Sims's design skills for producing gynecological instruments also secured his legacy. He patented, manufactured, and sold the instruments that he used—speculums, cannulas, and syringes—to provide the gynecological community tools to enlarge the cervical os, to dilate, to make incisions, and to insert pessaries. These decisions to name and to patent instruments, not to mention to develop a double-bladed speculum now known as a Sims' speculum, kept his name and his association with gynecological surgery alive after his death. Other gynecologists capitalized on Sims's initiatives and began to manufacture and to sell their own syringes and cannulas for other physicians and would be home inseminators. For example, the American physician Edward Bliss Foote (1829–1905) saw the technique's money-making potential and began marketing a syringe for home AI use in 1870, and eighty-five years later, the physician Joan Malleson (1899–1956) designed an AI syringe that was manufactured by Allen & Hanburys (a British pharmaceutical company) in 1955.[11] Sims ensured his technological longevity in gynecology by providing clear descriptions of his experiments, tools, and procedures in his publications. However, it is impossible to evaluate his work without recognizing the enslaved women who non-consensually participated as his research subjects.

The technological history of AI remained static for decades after Sims published his description of it in 1866, though the circumstances in which it was used (either by physicians or at home) and the sperm used in the process (from the husband, an anonymous donor, a known donor, or a mixture of husband and donor sperm) varied significantly. The tools—a syringe, cannula, and small canister or jar for the semen—stayed the same. Additionally, the semen had to be fresh, at least until the establishment of sperm banks in the 1950s allowed for sperm to be frozen ahead of time (see below).

Some physicians tried adding other apparatuses to these basic elements. The physician Joseph Gérard (1834–1898), who publicized AI techniques in France through the defense of his thesis on "artificial fecundation" at the University of Paris in 1885, designed and manufactured his own syringe and cannula, and promoted his innovative "portable fecundation stirrup." As Bridget Gurtler observes, by "using portable stirrups, science literally entered the bedroom with the physician so that the procedure could be performed post-coitus by attaching the stirrups to the bed."[12] The normalization of AI in US and European gynecology sparked different reactions among members of the medical community, and Gérard played a key role in debates about it. For example, he noted in *Nouvelles causes de stérilité dans les deux sexes* (1888) that the "artificial" part of AI could benefit society (as a sign of modernity) or could harm it (if donor AI threatened the association of masculinity and fertility). "It was the man-made nature of the syringe as a replacement for marriage and sexual relationships with men, and the implied 'unnaturalness' of the act when compared to the sexual act that caused the most consternation," Gurtler writes.[13] And until the timing of ovulation was confirmed in the 1920s and publicized in the 1930s, calculation of the best time in the menstrual cycle for AI treatment—syringe, cannula, stirrups, and all—was guesswork.

As the use of AI was often kept secret, due to embarrassment on the married couple's part, the illegality of the treatment, or its being forbidden by the Roman Catholic Church from 1897 onward, reports of children conceived with AI were publicly received with mixtures of curiosity, anger, or even disgust at medical interference with the natural process of sexual intercourse.[14] Professor William H. Pancoast (1834–1897) at Jefferson Medical College in

Philadelphia is a case in point. Pancoast used donor sperm from one of his students to impregnate the wife of an affluent acquaintance with the acquaintance's (but not his wife's) consent in 1884. According to Addison Davis Hard (d. 1931), who was Pancoast's student at the time and wrote about the case in a letter to the editor of *The Medical World* in 1909, the sperm came from "the best-looking member of the class." The husband had likely become sterile after a gonorrhea infection, and the wife never knew the true identity of her child's father. Scholars who reviewed the case in 1965 and again in 1997 speculated that Hard himself was the sperm donor, as he had recently met the twenty-five-year-old man in New York City, and there was a twenty-five-year difference between the alleged event and Hard's letter.[15] What really happened in 1884 is impossible to know, but the persistence of this letter in the history of medicine illustrates ongoing interest in the possibility that AI could disguise genetic parentage and that physicians and husbands would deceive women if it served their own interests in perpetuating family heritage.

But such cases of trickery were rare. By the 1910s, technology-assisted AI with husband or donor sperm was old news for US and European gynecologists. For example, in the United States, Dr. Eliza Mosher (1846–1928) wrote an article in 1912 advocating AI as both "proper and peculiarly adapted to women in medicine," and Dr. Robert Latou Dickinson (1861–1950) used his inaugural speech as the newly elected president of the American Gynecological Society in 1920 to promote research on "artificial impregnation." In 1920s Germany and Switzerland, AI for both humans and animals was a popular topic of discussion, though few gynecologists, including Dr. Hermann Rohleder (1866–1934), would admit to using it. Rohleder would perform AI with donor sperm only for patients with azoospermia and for desperate, "high quality" couples— the quality of whom he determined himself.[16]

If a couple wanted to try the process on their own and had access to medical literature, they could use a book like the Enid, Oklahoma-based physician Dr. Frank P. Davis's *Impotency, Sterility, and Artificial Impregnation* (1917). Davis (1868–1932) argued that by teaching people how to do AI themselves, "we overcome the aesthetical objections to artificial fecundation, and thus are enabled to relieve many cases of barrenness."[17] However, if a couple wanted a physician's assistance, they could arrange postcoital AI, a process that the Dutch physician Dr. Theodoor H. van de Velde (1873–1937) described in his 1929 book *Fertility and Sterility in Marriage*. Van de Velde adapted the process from the Sims-Huhner test, which had an identical first step.

First, the couple had intercourse while the doctor waited nearby. After ejaculation, they would summon the doctor, who would immediately scoop out the ejaculate into a spray device. The doctor would then perform AI: "The portio (of the vagina) must then be grasped by a tenaculum forceps, the cannula of the spray passed up through the cervix until its extremity is at least above the interior os, and then a little of the seminal fluid should be slowly injected into the uterus." Then, "the cannula should be left motionless for a few minutes, and then very slowly retracted, the portio released, the speculum removed and the woman put into the horizontal position with as little movement as possible, and kept quiet in bed for the day." Alternatively, the couple could have intercourse at home with a condom, then bring the ejaculate-filled condom to the doctor's office where AI would then take place. Van de Velde rather grandly called this process *Coitus Condomatus*.[18] It is doubtful that the term was widespread, but evidence from the United States and Europe shows that the practice itself certainly was.

Stem Pessaries, Cotton, and Sexual Positions

After AI with a syringe and cannula was regularized among physicians in Europe and the United States, they began in the 1910s and 1920s to experiment with methods for improving the likelihood that sperm would reach the uterus and fertilize an oocyte. Some recommended that women simply lie down with their pelvis and legs elevated for several hours after sexual intercourse so that the semen would not leak out when they stood. Van de Velde described how some German gynecologists combined this natural use of gravity with a cervical cap (*Portiokappe* in German) or stem pessary. For example, a Dr. Pust recommended in 1914 that "sufficient seminal fluid should be deposited in one of the portio cap pessaries and the pessary then at once placed in position on the extremity of the cervix," then left alone for twenty-four hours. However, Van de Velde considered that length of time "too long an interval," due to the possibility of discomfort and infection.[19]

To take another example, the Munich-based gynecologist Dr. Max Nassauer (1869–1931) encouraged patients to use a pessary that he designed, the Fructulet, which had a flat base to occlude the vaginal canal and a stem that kept the cervix open so that sperm were not blocked from reaching the uterus. Nassauer's Fructulet was subject to wide debate among members of the German medical community. Another gynecologist, the Stuttgart-based Dr. Hermann Fehling (1847–1925), dilated a woman's cervix with a sound (elongated metal instrument) and, after intercourse, inserted an aseptic glass tube that would stay in place for three days, which Fehling would then irrigate each day in an attempt to prevent infection. Van de Velde recommended that women with uterine displacement, especially retroflexion, could wear stem pessaries to correct those displacements. However, inserting a foreign object

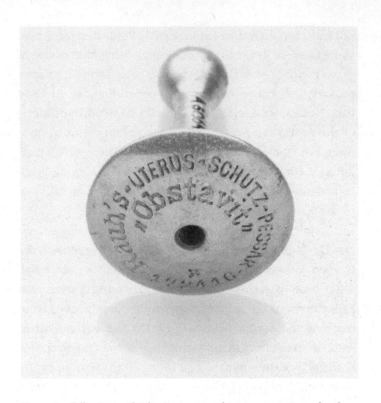

Figure 2 Following artificial insemination, physicians sometimes placed a uterine pessary like Rauh's "Obstavit" (c. 1925–1935) to keep the semen inside the female patient and to improve chances that sperm would reach the uterus. *Source:* Courtesy the Board of Trustees of the Science Museum, CC BY-NC-SA 4.0.

in the vaginal canal and keeping it there for several days could easily lead to infection—not to mention significant discomfort.[20]

In addition to methods that required one or more visits to a physician, Van de Velde described inexpensive, low- or no-tech methods for home use. Married couples who could not afford physician-assisted AI "may make use of such more or less primitive methods as saturation of cotton wool, of tampons or of sprays in the seminal ejaculate and their [subsequent] insertion into the vagina."[21] Finally, he put forward the idea that sexual intercourse with the woman on top instead of on her back could improve the chance of conception. Though there is no evidence that sexual positioning had any effect, simply changing positions required no technological or physician assistance, and it was certainly the least expensive and least dangerous method among the many ineffective methods that Van de Velde proposed.

Finally, some physicians in the late nineteenth and early twentieth centuries turned their attention to the health of sperm. Without spermatic analysis and absent a clear exterior marker like impotence, male infertility could be hard to diagnose, much less treat. There was also no direct link between sexually transmitted infections like syphilis and gonorrhea and infertility. Even though Salvarsan (arsphenamine) as a treatment for syphilis was available in some countries starting in 1909, not all men had access to it, and it contained arsenic. Children could still be conceived by parents infected with gonorrhea and syphilis, which led to serious conditions like blindness.[22] Most physicians did not delve into scientific sperm research, but those who practiced AI passed on folk wisdom to potential donors: for example, testicles should be kept cool, as overheated testicles could damage sperm. They also encouraged donors to wear boxer shorts instead of briefs to allow the freer movement of the testicles and to immerse their testicles in cool water from time to time.[23]

A few researchers made advances in spermatic analysis. The National Committee on Maternal Health (NCMH), established by Robert Latou Dickinson in New York in 1923, supported the research of Gerald L. Moench on sperm. Instead of focusing on motility, as J. Marion Sims and Max Huhner had, Moench centered his energies on describing sperm morphology and investigating the relationship of morphology to male fertility. So, the first diagnostic tool to be used in the detection of male infertility was the "spermatozoa count," or sperm count, developed in 1929, made possible by "imaging technologies, such as electron microscopes and other devices, [which] create[d] new opportunities to produce scientific knowledge about sperm." Examining and counting sperm under a microscope helped a physician diagnose if a patient had inactive or abnormally moving sperm, azoospermia (an absence of sperm), or oligospermia (inadequate sperm).

Azoospermia could be obstructive (when the route from the testes to the epididymis [small ducts holding sperm] is congenitally missing or blocked) or nonobstructive (a complete absence of germ cells). Unfortunately, there were no reputable treatments available to revive or to rejuvenate sperm.[24]

Due to sperm's association with sex and venereal disease, though, only a few other researchers followed Moench and others in their quest to understand sperm for much of the twentieth century. The Roman Catholic Church's restrictions on masturbation, even for a diagnostic purpose, hindered research in countries in which physician associations adhered to its strictures. So Mexican doctors, for example, studied sperm only from semen obtained immediately after heterosexual intercourse in the framework of a Sims-Huhner test.[25]

The sperm-related experiments conducted in the 1930s were few and far between. A rare example is from a clinical urology professor at Columbia University, who catheterized the ejaculatory ducts of an infertile intending father and then used a syringe to inject semen from a healthy blood relative into his seminal vesicle. "By this method," wrote C. Travers Stepita (1897–1982), "the opportunity for impregnation is afforded in a perfectly natural and aesthetic manner," if the man could somehow forget that a relative's semen had just been injected into his groin.[26] This method does not seem to have been successful, as it appears only once in medical literature—no doubt much to future patients' relief.

Sperm-oriented research was revived in the 1950s and centered on pooling and centrifuging techniques. For the latter, Drs. John Rock (1890–1984) and Frederick M. Hanson developed a method of centrifuging semen to increase the sperm concentrations of subpar ejaculates by spinning them, pouring off excess liquid, adding Locke's solution (a salt solution), and repeating the process until the sediment was concentrated and ready for insemination. Edmond J. Farris was another early researcher and advocate of this method. He estimated that when the ejaculate of around 4.5 cubic centimeters (cc) was centrifuged to a volume of 1 cc, the sperm counts increased from 44 to 113 million per cc and the number of active spermatozoa increased from 18 to 33 million per cc. For the pooling technique, physicians would mix together several ejaculations from a husband with a low sperm count, sometimes taken over a period of weeks. Another method was to ask the husband to ejaculate into separate containers and simply use AI with the better specimen.[27] These advancements were relatively low-tech but appeared to have some positive effect on achieving pregnancy among small numbers of patients. More high-tech advancements took place in the area of freezing (see later in this chapter), and other physicians became interested in tackling fertility problems from an alternative angle: hormones.

Hormones

The identification of hormones, their sources, and their functions from the mid-1910s onward intrigued physicians in all specialties, including gynecologists. Endocrinology quickly became an active research field, and gynecologists paid close attention to (and sometimes contributed to) research on how hormones affected reproduction and fertility. Estrogen was isolated in 1923, and progesterone was isolated in 1924. The existence of gonadotropins (hormones that produce gametes in the ovary or testes) was discovered in 1926 when scientists in the United States and Germany demonstrated that ovulation was a response of the ovaries to a hormonal communication from another gland. In 1927, a German gynecologist named Bernhard Zondek (1891–1966) discovered that the anterior lobe of the pituitary gland was responsible for the production of gonadotropins. Then, in the same year, he isolated human chorionic gonadotropin (hCG)—the substance that leads to the formation of the corpus luteum (the progesterone-secreting tissue that forms immediately after ovulation)—but no one knew if taking it as a supplement would help with fertility.[28]

That lack of knowledge did not stop physicians and pharmaceutical companies from capitalizing on Zondek's findings. Once hormones were isolated from other elements of the human body, physicians in the United States,

United Kingdom, and German- and Dutch-speaking Europe began to offer gonadotropins as supplements to patients in the early 1930s. The preparations were very expensive, and their effectiveness was uncertain. In the book *Human Sterility* (1934), the Boston-based gynecologist Samuel R. Meaker promoted unproven hormonal treatments, including preparations from the pituitary, thyroid, and ovary glands. These treatments were often available in the United States and United Kingdom without a prescription.[29]

Van de Velde, the Dutch gynecologist, outlined analogous ideas that his fellow practitioners tried with their patients in the 1920s and early 1930s. In Dutch- and German-speaking Europe, hormone supplements were marketed under brand names such as Ovoglandol (ovarian hormone), Menformon (follicular), Thyreoidin, Thyroxin (thyroidal), Adrenalin (adrenal), and Prolan (pituitary lobe). For the specific problem of "genital infantilism," there were "doses of ovarian or other (pluriglandular) preparations; diathermy (radiant heat) and vibromassage." He proposed placing substances in the vagina that would speed the movement of semen into the uterus, such as "blood serum, solutions of albumin and glycerine, and weak alkaline solutions, especially in combination with carbonic acid."[30] Men could try testicular compounds, yohimbin and yohistrin compounds, and muiracithin compounds. Needless to say, none of these supplements had any effect. Other technologies held more promise for improving the chance of pregnancy.

Surgery, Insufflation, and Salpingograms

Along with ovulatory abnormalities, cervical factors, and spermatic absence or deficiency, blockages in the fallopian tubes were a common source of fertility problems. Surgeons could attempt to remove these blockages via a high-risk procedure called a salpingostomy (opening the fallopian tubes surgically), which was first attempted in 1889. Women became pregnant after this surgery at a rate of only 7 percent (US) and 8–10 percent (UK).[31] Father and son physicians William L. Estes, Sr. (1855–1940) and William L. Estes, Jr. (1895–1971), both practicing in Bethlehem, Pennsylvania, developed another surgical procedure that connected the ovaries directly to the uterus on one or both sides, bypassing the fallopian tubes. Then, ovulation could take place directly in the uterus. The Estes operation never became popular among gynecological surgeons, likely due to its still-low success rate compared to the salpingostomy. In a 1910 article, Estes Sr. stated that out of forty operations, he knew of two pregnancies and one live birth. Estes Jr.'s investigations into its historical use revealed two live births after twenty-seven operations from 1895 to 1924, and his decision to not treat anyone over the age of thirty indicated his belief that it was best suited for younger patients. After news of Louise Brown's birth via IVF in 1978 (chapter 3), there was a brief revival of interest in the procedure, but it faded again after lower-risk IVF procedures became widespread.[32]

In the 1910s, two European gynecologists turned their attention from reparatory surgery techniques to diagnostic tools, and in doing so made major advances in fertility diagnostics. Drs. Isidor C. Rubin (1883–1958) in Vienna and G. Le Lorier in Paris designed the nonsurgical technique of insufflation contemporaneously. Rubin began his experiments in 1914 with injecting a colloidal silver solution (Collargol) into the wombs of deceased mammals and women, to see if it would improve X-ray diagnoses. World War I interrupted both of their research programs, and Rubin escaped to New York City. In 1919, he revived his experiments on living women with a different set of substances. He drove oxygen and carbonic acid gas into the tubal duct from the uterus with a machine called a tubal insufflator combined with a manometer (an instrument that measures the pressure of gases or vapors), which showed and regulated the necessary degree of pressure. Insufflation pushed gas into a woman's uterus to inflate it, which then would show the amount of blockage in the fallopian tubes. The amount of pressure that indicated clear fallopian tubes varied according to how many children the woman had birthed, and the pressure itself could also remove some tissue blockages by force. The pressure measurement was expressed on a graphing instrument called a kymograph, which recorded the changes in pelvic pressure that the manometer measured.[33]

In 1925, Rubin presented his machines and technique at a meeting of the Section of Obstetrics and Gynecology, Royal Society of Medicine in the United Kingdom. By the end of the decade, Dr. Sidney Forsdike (1874–1942), a surgeon at the Soho Hospital for Women in London, developed an analogous process using an oil-based solution (lipiodol, an oil containing 10 percent iodine) and X-rays. The lipiodol was injected into the uterus with a rubber bulb attached to a Tykos-brand manometer with a fluorescent face. The fluorescence was necessary because the tests were administered in a dark room in order for the gynecologist and the X-ray technician to see fluid move through the X-rays properly. After the diagnostic session, the lipiodol could remain in the pelvic cavity up to six months, causing irritation. Forsdike's method was called a salpingogram or hysterosalpingogram and identified the location of the blockage more precisely than insufflation.[34]

The establishment of insufflation and the salpingogram as techniques and the creation of the machines used to execute them had a profound effect on fertility diagnostics. As Van de Velde put it, "by means of insufflation and salpingograms, it has become possible to ascertain and exactly locate such causes of feminine sterility as

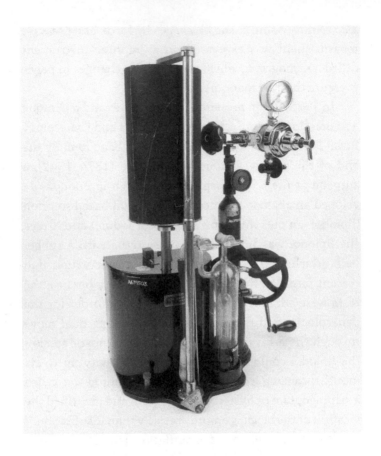

Figure 3 Physicians used insufflation machines for both diagnostic and therapeutic purposes: to determine blockages in the fallopian tubes and to clear them. Utero-tubal insufflation apparatus, without some items, made by Becker, from Italian Hospital in London, American make, 1928. *Source:* Courtesy the Board of Trustees of the Science Museum, CC BY-NC-SA 4.0.

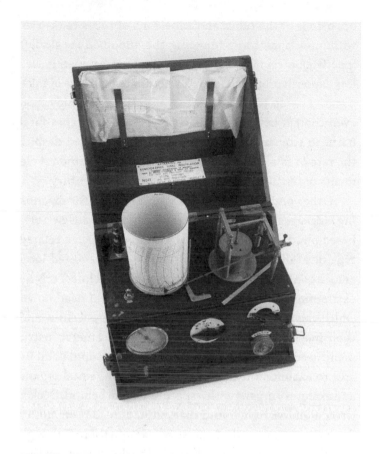

Figure 4 Insufflation apparatus, made by Kelvin, Bottomley, & Baird Limited, Glasgow, Scotland, c. 1935 1945. The kymograph with its stylus and rotating cylinder is visible at the front. *Source:* Courtesy the Board of Trustees of the Science Museum, CC BY-NC-SA 4.0.

occlusions of the tubes and adhesions of tubes to ovaries" without a laparotomy (opening the abdomen surgically). Insufflation remained more widely used because it was less expensive, but it had an unfortunate high rate of false negatives—up to 37 percent in a 1949–1952 study.[35] So even though both methods could potentially cause fatal harm to women via embolism or infection, and despite the rate of false negatives, their use became standard elements of fertility medicine for the next half-century.

Other physicians tinkered with methods for diagnosing blockages in the fallopian tubes. In 1939, a New York–based physician called Albert Decker developed a related type of examination, the culdoscopy, that required local anesthesia but not surgery. A patient would kneel on the examining table and place her forearms and head down, which raised her bottom in the air. The physician would then insert a culdoscope (a long, pointed metal instrument used to view the pelvic cavity) and cannula and be able to examine the fallopian tubes, other genital organs, and excretory organs with a speculum from behind. Decker wrote that "we have found that patients readily submit to the examination and to repeated examinations," though how they actually felt is unknown. The director of the Hospital de la Mujer in Mexico City, Alfonso Gutiérrez Nájar (1930–2014), mastered the technique in the 1940s and established a training center to teach others how to use it. The culdoscopy did not replace insufflation or laparotomy but provided physicians an alternative—perhaps less painful but still uncomfortable—form of diagnosing the same problem.[36]

However advanced surgically based diagnostic methods became, though, they were not infertility cures. Gynecologists from the 1910s through the 1950s focused on blockages in the fallopian tubes and paid less attention to other factors involved in fertility, such as ovulatory abnormalities, cervical factors, and sperm deficiency. Other findings in the 1920s, such as the timing of ovulation, would add to knowledge about the reproductive system but would not cure infertility either.

The Timing of Ovulation

Another avenue toward improving fertility was determining the timing of ovulation. Once this information was available, sexual intercourse and/or AI could be timed in order to give the sperm the best possible chance of reaching that singular monthly egg. In a 1905 experiment, Van de Velde made inroads into the problem by using an armpit thermometer to measure women's temperatures during their monthly menstrual cycles. He observed that women's temperatures rose and fell in regular patterns throughout the month. He thought that ovulation occurred at the lowest temperature point of the cycle and was indicated by a sudden rise in temperature but could not confirm his conclusions.[37]

Confirmation of Van de Velde's speculation was not determined until Kyusaku Ogino and Hermann H. Knaus published their research results a generation later in 1923 and 1929, respectively. Ogino began his research into ovulation in May 1919, and he became familiar with the German-language research on the subject with the help of a German Catholic priest who tutored him. He studied the cycles of sixty-five women patients at Niigata University Hospital and determined that ovulation happened within twelve to sixteen days before women's next menstrual period. He first published his results in a Japanese medical journal in February 1923, and by 1928, he had authored twenty-six papers on ovulation. However, his work was not known outside the Japanese-speaking world until he traveled to Germany to give a speech in 1928. One of his articles was published in a German gynecological journal in November 1930, and his results compared closely to those of Knaus. Following the article's publication, Knaus sent Ogino a letter congratulating him on his findings.[38]

Knaus himself was an assistant physician at the Universitäts-Frauenklinik (University Women's Clinic) in Graz, Austria, when he began his research on ovulation in rabbits and later collaborated with a colleague to see if his hypotheses were correct about ovulation in women. Knaus first presented his work at the German Society of

Gynecology conference in Leipzig in 1929, and he wrote an article for the *Münchener Medizinische Wochenschrift* (*Munich Medical Weekly*) based on his presentation, proclaiming: "An egg cell is only fertile for a few hours, which means that women with regular, four-week cycles can no longer conceive in the first 10 days and from the 18th day of the cycle onward at the latest."[39] Both men found that women ovulated approximately fifteen days before their next menstrual period began. So, for the best chance of pregnancy, sexual intercourse should occur on that day (Knaus) or the two days on either side of it (Ogino). Their discoveries were based on the daylong survival of the egg, the fact that sperm survived up to five days in the reproductive tract after sexual intercourse, studying patients' six-month-long menstrual cycle records, and averaging the longest and shortest cycles.[40] Their work has provided the foundation for both fertility and contraceptive timing methods ever since. As their findings were so similar, ovulation timing was named after both of them.

After Ogino-Knaus timing methods were published in multiple languages in the early 1930s, especially through Catholic advocates such as Leo J. Latz (1903–1994) in the United States and Johannes N. J. Smulders (1872–1939) in the Netherlands, manufacturers designed calendars and clocks to help identify ovulation timing. The problem with depending on time alone was that any number of bodily occurrences—breastfeeding, menopause, travel,

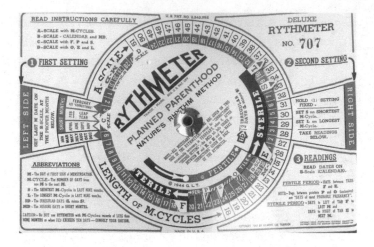

Figure 5 After medical confirmation of the timing of ovulation, manufacturers created devices to help track menstrual cycles. One of these was the Rhythmeter fertility planner, distributed by Planned Parenthood in 1944. *Source:* Courtesy Center for the History of Medicine, Countway Library of Medicine, Harvard University.

stress, and amenorrhea among them—could interfere with menstrual regularity. However, there are other physiological indicators that improve the reliability of timing methods: when ovulation is about to occur, body temperature rises between two-tenths and one degree above its preovulatory resting state. The basal body temperature (BBT) test, which is ideally conducted soon after rising in the morning, became popular in the late 1930s because it was inexpensive and easy to perform, and it increased public knowledge of ovulation timing.[41]

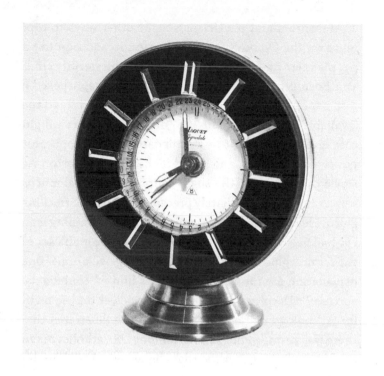

Figure 6 Another of these menstrual tracking devices was the Gynodate fertility clock, designed by Walter Thiele and manufactured by the Swiss clock manufacturer Jaquet in 1958. *Source:* Courtesy Museum of Contraception and Reproduction, Vienna.

Inventors and physicians sought other ways to capitalize on the Ogino-Knaus discoveries. In addition to paper planners and clocks, the director of the sterility clinic at a Boston hospital, Dr. Joseph B. Doyle, repurposed a test paper coated with glucose oxidase called Tes-Tape (available commercially in 1957) to measure cervical glucose levels, attached it to a cardboard tampon applicator, packaged it in a kit, and called it the Fertility Testor. As Doyle thought that "the sugar content of cervical mucus was . . . highest immediately preceding ovulation, tracking glucose levels could act as simple test for determining if an egg had been released." However, "the relative inefficacy of the cervical glucose method for predicting ovulation is one explanation for the Fertility Testor's limited commercial success."[42] Despite its lack of staying power on the fertility technology market, Doyle's invention illustrated that there was strong public interest among US Catholics for an ovulation tracking method that aligned with the Church's teachings.

Ovulation and AI: Combining Methods

Beginning in the early 1930s, physicians started to time AI treatments to coincide with ovulation to increase their chances of success. If the fertility problem was with the man's sperm (physicians in the United States, United

Kingdom, Mexico, Israel, Taiwan, and elsewhere only accepted heterosexual married couples for treatment at the time), physicians used donor sperm or mixed donor sperm with the husband's sperm to make any potential child's real parentage unknown. "Separating biological and social paternity went against centuries of effort by the [Roman Catholic] Church and the state to establish clear lines of paternity," and the mixed-sperm method also preserved the husband's sense of masculinity in the face of male factor infertility. The thinking behind this practice was as follows: the fact that a child *could* be his—even if it almost certainly was not—was less likely to challenge existing emotional bonds between him and his wife, him and his future child(ren), or his sense of his own virility.[43]

Physicians shared their methods for donor selection and AI with each other in print. Their methods sometimes included technologies outside normal clinical practice. To take one example, Robert Latou Dickinson "expected a husband providing semen for the insemination of his wife to produce 'a friction specimen about an hour before the appointed time' and to keep it 'warm but not hot, under a warm water bag or in a thermos bottle.'" To take another, "in the 1950s, Dr. Sophia Kleegman (1901–1971), a New York City practitioner who learned artificial insemination from Dickinson in 1931, relied on a taxi service to deliver fresh semen from her donors to her office, keeping the donor away from the place of insemination altogether."[44]

In 1969, Dr. Alan Guttmacher (1898–1974) outlined the procedures that he had used for AI since 1943. He accepted only married couples into his program and preferred married medical students or young doctors as donors. The donor would masturbate into a "clean, wide-necked bottle or jar" and deliver the specimen immediately to Guttmacher, who then liquefied it, diluted it, divided it into 1.2 cc glass ampules, froze it, and rethawed it as needed. For the insemination process itself, Guttmacher aspirated the sperm sample into a syringe with a cannula at the end. He then placed the cannula into the patient's vagina "and by intermittent pressure on the syringe plunger simulating the ejaculatory, expulsive mechanism of normal male orgasm, its contents spurted at the cervix in three or four thrusts." The patient would then lie still for twenty minutes, place a small piece of cotton over the vaginal opening to block leakage, and then return home.[45] The process, with the exception of the imitation thrusting, had changed little from Sims to Van de Velde, from Mosher to Guttmacher. Sperm banks would not change insemination procedures, but they would alter how sperm was stored and accessed, and whom it came from.

Sperm Banking

Long-term tissue and body product banking, specifically sperm banking, was a technological infrastructure important to expanding the reach of AI and making IVF viable (embryo and egg banking is discussed in chapter 3). Finding the appropriate media in which the body products would be best preserved was also important. Sperm banking began in the United States after a fertility clinic opened at the University of Iowa in 1952. Researchers there found that "slow freezing of glycerol-treated sperm on dry ice was the most successful in maintaining post-thaw motility," ensuring a survival rate of 60–78 percent.[46] The first Iowa experiments with frozen sperm (whether the sperm was from husbands or donors is unclear) resulted in four live births in 1954. Following their initial successes, Jerome K. Sherman (b. 1925) and Raymond J. Bunge discovered a liquid nitrogen–vapor freezing method that "could not only be cooled much more quickly than in air but would also freeze and store samples at very low temperatures (−190 to −196° C)."[47] As semen did not deteriorate at such a low temperature, it became the most popular method for sperm banking for the next several decades. Cryopreservation was then practiced on a small scale by US physicians in the 1960s and early 1970s. The development of cryopreservation as a technology in the 1950s did not alone force a change in sperm donation practices or the medical practice of AI in individual clinics, since a social stigma against using donor sperm remained present in US culture. Sophia Kleegman was the lone US physician advocating for a centrally organized sperm bank management system, first in 1953 and throughout the 1960s, to take the burden of decision-making away from doctors. As Kara Swanson notes, "the new technology of cryopreservation was not sufficient to overcome medical resistance to organized supplies of semen."[48]

That resistance would not last forever, though. The first public sperm bank opened in Denmark in 1967, and the first commercial bank opened in the United States in 1971, offering an opportunity for entrepreneurs to provide those concerned about their fertility (particularly men undergoing chemotherapy) with a form of "fertility insurance." Whether the sperm was purchased or donated, most fertility specialists continued to prefer fresh sperm, and many also selected the donor themselves in cases where a husband was infertile. "The first commercial banks . . . [offered] frozen sperm stored in tanks of liquid nitrogen, but they struggled against the perception that frozen-and-thawed sperm resulted in lower rates of conception than 'fresh' sperm."[49]

As commercial sperm banks became more widespread throughout the mid-1970s, they began to take over the process of donor selection from physicians. Additionally, the HIV/AIDS crisis of the 1980s created the need to test and freeze sperm before use, physically separating the physician from donors and their emissions. Few if any physicians had the capacity to store semen using liquid nitrogen on their own. After six American women between 1986 and 1989 became infected with HIV due to insemination with infected fresh sperm, "most physicians had little choice but to turn to commercial banks, which had the infrastructure necessary to freeze sperm, quarantine the samples, ship them, and monitor donors for months and months on end."[50]

As the use of fresh sperm in clinic settings declined, so did the common practice of donor selection by physicians and in-office inseminations. From the 1990s onward, sperm banks began the practice of soliciting donors on their own, bypassing sales to physicians and selling sperm directly to clients. Given that change in consumer dynamics, those clients could perform insemination at home on their own or could ask a physician to assist them, but the physician was no longer central to the process. Furthermore, "once sperm banks transitioned to purchasing semen from donors as the major part of their business . . . a bank could build up a breadth and depth of inventory."[51] The establishment of commercial sperm banking had ramifications across the growing fertility services and body product industry. Whereas artificial insemination was once a secretive if not-unknown procedure conducted in medical settings, the establishment of commercial sperm banks cut out the physician as a broker, shifted the power of sperm choice from the physician to the consumer, and turned the buying and selling of sperm into a money-making enterprise.

In the present, cryobanking has developed into a large-scale industry that "not only stores product but also procures, screens, and manipulates it." Sperm banks look for donors who "are generally expected to be tall and college educated." For example, the Danish clinic Cryos leans heavily on the idea that its donors are passing on Viking genes: "The Viking metaphor simultaneously reiterates the donors' gendering as masculine and becomes a guarantor for the potency of the sperm." Some banks structure client access to donor information in tiers—the more that potential recipients pay, the more information about the donor the banks share with them.[52]

The characteristics of a good sperm donor are not visible to the naked eye, though. "The majority of potential sperm donors are interestingly not turned down because they lack the appearance-based qualities that interest sperm buyers, but simply because they are 'bad freezers.'" In other words, their semen must survive the technological processes of becoming "technosemen" (chapter 6) to be salable to potential buyers. Successful sperm donors masturbate to provide their donations and manage periods of abstinence according to schedules that the bank determines, and one measurement of sperm quality is "its statistical success rate as determined by the number of successful pregnancies from the bank." That success lies in part with their sperm's receptivity to freezing and thawing and in part with donors following the rules governing their out-of-clinic sexual behavior.[53]

The characteristics of a good sperm donor are not visible to the naked eye.

Sperm donation practices in China provide a useful comparison to donation practices in the United States, illustrating how analogous technological processes manifest in countries with different political frameworks, population policies, and technical infrastructures. After the Cultural Revolution ended in 1976, medical laboratories had become derelict and doctors had had to rebuild them and their own skills from scratch. Lu Guangxiu, for example, learned "how to freeze sperm using egg yolk and glycerol in 1980 . . . to have access to sperm in the laboratory for in vitro research purposes." By 1984, she had established China's first sperm bank, and one year later, she traveled to the United States to learn "laboratory procedures such as sperm washing, determination of the level of maturity of an egg, culture medium preparation, and embryo morphology assessment." Her efforts, combined with those of Zhang Lizhu (1925–2016) on egg retrieval, led to the birth of the country's first IVF-assisted baby in 1988. Assisted reproductive technologies were legalized in 2003, and the country is now "one of the most strictly regulated ART sectors in the world, as it has had to conform to national family planning regulations."[54]

Recruiters at present-day Chinese sperm banks solicit college-educated donors by visiting university cities in vans. They hand out flyers and canvas in university dorms and on social media to solicit donors. Each van has a mobile sperm bank kit in a large yellow box, which holds "a microscope, vials for preserving sperm, petri dishes for the bacterial smears that each stored sample is subjected to, a few white coats, latex gloves, hairnets, surgical masks, and a stethoscope."[55] After recruitment, donors are given supplies and instructions on preparing for donation in a private room at a clinic—using disinfectant, a sample cup, and some cotton pads—and they bring their mobile phones to play pornographic videos, as clinics provide no erotic stimulation. They are paid more if their sperm is usable and less if it is not.

Following the donation, clinicians place the semen samples into a Julabo warm-water bath machine to liquefy them. Lab workers check the viscosity of the sample, count the number of sperm cells in a square on a slide, examine the semen, and estimate the percentage of motile sperm. Samples are prepared for cryopreservation by mixing them with a portion of cryoprotectant made of glycerol and egg yolk. The sample is injected into vials and labeled. The sample vials are checked for bacteria, then "placed into a ThermoFisher controlled-rate freezer that brings the temperature of samples down. . . . Once the freezer has rather loudly clicked and buzzed its way to well-below freezing temperatures, vials are taken out and transferred into a cylindrical cryotank's trays, which have been pulled out of the tank's liquid nitrogen using a steel rod and gloves."[56] The trays are then replaced in the tank. By then, the donors are on their way home.

The differences between China and the United States are notable in how clinics handle sperm after donation. Chinese donors may provide sperm to a maximum of five different women, in order to minimize the chance that half-siblings will become sexual partners without knowing it. As a result, sperm banks have chronic shortages and must constantly seek new donors. Further, sperm donation is conducted through a double-blind system, which "is a defining feature of sperm banking in China."[57] The doctor, the social parents, and the child never know who the donor is, the donor will never know who they are, and, often, the parents do not tell the child about the child's parentage.

The examples of American and Chinese sperm banks and use of donor sperm illustrate how similar technologies and processes operate in markedly dissimilar ways. On the one hand, in China, restrictions on quantities and qualities of sperm use, the routinization of donation and use, and the anonymization of the actors involved standardizes the process of donation and requires that child-seekers trust state actors to decide what sperm is best for them. On the other hand, in the United States, child-seekers have greater agency over the sperm they select; they can increase payments to clinics for more information about donors; and future children may or may not have the legal right to learn their genetic parentage. Each country's political structures and approaches to market regulation generally structure access to, and use of, fertility technology.

There have been a wide range of technologies used in the pursuit of pregnancy and childbirth. Many of these require medical assistance or approval, and their use depends on the physician's willingness to accept a patient for treatment and to use a tool like tubal insufflation. Other technologies, like the cannula and syringe, are usable either with or without professional assistance. The next chapter focuses on a method that is possible only with extensive medical support: IVF. IVF places the process of child-seeking squarely into the realm of medical systems, requiring much funding, patience, and time. It also expands procreative options beyond the heterosexual childless couple targeted for AI in the pre-IVF era. IVF and its associated technologies, including surrogacy, can make children—either with donated gametes or one's own—possible for a wide range of individuals and families.

IVF AND ITS SUCCESSORS

From the 1860s forward, technological development in the area of fertility proceeded along two paths: diagnostics and treatments. While innovation in diagnostic technologies like insufflation remained relatively static for decades, a small number of obstetricians, gynecologists, and embryologists started pursuing treatments in the 1960s that eventually revolutionized treatment for those desiring pregnancy: in vitro ("in glass") fertilization, or IVF. As many ailments (including appendicitis, ovarian cysts, abdominal or pelvic surgery complications, endometriosis, or pelvic inflammatory disease) could easily damage the fallopian tubes, it is no wonder that IVF developed to work around a specific and particularly intractable type of infertility—blocked or otherwise damaged fallopian tubes. This chapter traces the history of IVF, the additional procedures that expanded its reach, its spread around the world, and the technological infrastructures surrounding it.

Experiments with IVF as a technique and the technologies necessary to make it possible began on animals. A professor at the University of Vienna, Leopold Schenk (1840–1902), published the earliest recorded attempt at an IVF procedure using rabbit ova in 1878. Dr. Gregory Pincus (1903–1967), best known for his research on the hormonal birth control pill, successfully conducted IVF on rabbits in 1936 and 1937. However, Pincus was denied tenure at Harvard University and had to build his own research institute in Worcester, Massachusetts, without the consistent support of a university. Pincus's IVF research slowed, given that he had to move his laboratory and then fundraise to keep his research program afloat.[1]

Human fertility specialists, including John Rock, saw the potential application of IVF animal experiments for their patients. Rock read about Pincus's experiments and decided to try human IVF himself at the Free Hospital for Women in Boston, where he directed the sterility clinic.[2] Rock and his colleague Dr. Arthur T. Hertig (1904–1990), along with his assistant, Miriam Menkin (1901–1992), conducted the earliest IVF experiments with human tissue in the Boston area in the 1940s. Although they had only partial success and never reached the point of implanting an embryo into a patient, their attempts to do so received extensive professional and media attention.

The next sections examine the Rock group's results in detail, before turning to the England-based research group whose efforts later manifested the first human birth via IVF.

Fertilization from the Outside: An Early Experiment

It was clear to Rock that the common practice of laparotomy (surgery to clear blockages in the fallopian tubes)—with its physiological complications and approximate 7 percent success rate—was not a viable method for curing infertility in most women. Developing a technique of in vitro fertilization would enable physicians to bypass damaged or blocked fallopian tubes by fertilizing an egg outside the body and then implanting it directly in the uterus. In vitro fertilization was not, then, a means of solving fertility problems, but a way to circumvent unfixable anatomical problems in order to make pregnancy possible.

Rock investigated the possibilities of IVF in two ways. First, he needed a more fine-grained understanding of the processes of conception, from fertilization to implantation in the uterus. While the Ogino-Knaus method of ovulation timing was widely known by the mid-1930s, and the "rhythm clinic" that Rock oversaw was devoted to teaching fertility (or, clandestinely, contraceptive) timing to Catholic patients, much less was known about the timing of the fertilized egg's movement to the uterus, its subsequent attachment to the uterine lining, and the development of the amniotic sac. To establish some basic facts about these processes, Rock and Hertig made a photographic study in 1941 of the initial stages of pregnancy using the remains of early pregnancies after hysterectomies. Patients participated in their experiments by planning to have intercourse shortly before the operation and then agreeing to donate their uterine tissue for medical study. Following the operation, which Rock performed, Hertig took the tissue into his laboratory to search for an ovum (unfertilized egg), fertilized egg, blastocyst (fertilized egg in early stages of cell division), conceptus (fertilized egg before implantation), or embryo (fertilized egg after implantation). If he found any of these, he transported them personally from Boston to the Carnegie Institution in Baltimore, where they were photographed and stored. The resulting articles provided evidence for the timing of these processes, which later researchers then used to time the extraction of an ovum for IVF.[3]

The second step in Rock's research was to investigate if an extracted ovum could, in fact, be fertilized outside the body. Rock and Menkin began a study in 1941 to track the timing of patient ovulation, in the hopes that they could rush patients to the hospital to extract eggs at just the right moment. That idea, along with an idea to remove eggs from the fallopian tubes surgically, was unsuccessful. Eventually, they experimented with eggs from patients who agreed to donate them while undergoing reproduction-related surgeries, fertilized those eggs with sperm from donors or leftover from AI treatments, and incubated them overnight. Menkin managed to fertilize an egg in vitro in February 1944, but the embryo lasted through only two cell divisions. She did so again in April, for a total of four ova fertilized from three patients. The publication of the results—including photographs by the Carnegie Institution staff member Chester Heuser, who also photographed the Hertig-Rock specimens—drew considerable public attention and speculation about the future of reproduction. Despite this widespread publicity, Rock abandoned the initial experiments in 1950 when he contemplated how long it would take to achieve a live birth via this process and turned his attention to the opposite: the suppression of fertility via the hormonal birth control pill.[4] A different group of researchers would tackle the next steps, including the placement of the fertilized egg in the uterus, a positive test for pregnancy, and live birth.

In Vitro Fertilization: Antecedents

IVF was built on the fertility-related discoveries from the last quarter of the nineteenth century to the first half of the twentieth century, including the function of reproductive

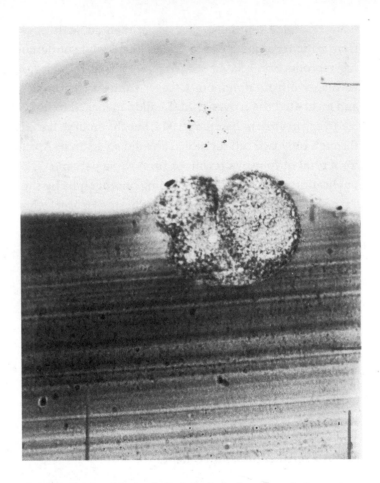

Figure 7 Egg found during the Rock-Hertig Study, still attached to endometrial tissue, c. 1945. *Source:* Courtesy Center for the History of Medicine, Countway Library of Medicine, Harvard University.

hormones, the timing of ovulation and implantation, the development of laparotomy and laparoscopy as surgical techniques, and the creation of an appropriate medium for the egg to grow. To become reality, IVF needed funding, technological know-how, the correct tools, and the right people with the right skills working together.

If the timing of natural ovulation could be determined with basal body temperature, as Ogino and Knaus first realized, some scientists thought that they could manifest ovulation artificially as well. Between 1949 and 1953, researchers in Rome and Geneva tried just that: they extracted and purified a human gonadotropin hormone from the urine of nuns and menopausal women that initiated ovulation, given to patients under the brand name Pergonal. Additionally, a new synthetic called Clomid (clomiphene citrate) that also initiated ovulation was discovered and tested at the same time.[5] Once the timing of ovulation could be regulated medically, physicians could plan the harvest of an egg for fertilization outside the womb. The company that produced Pergonal, Ares Serono, funded the Cambridge lab, a relationship that forged long-term financial links between the lab and the company.

The trio that would become famous for IVF research, Patrick Steptoe (a gynecologist), Robert Edwards (an embryologist), and Jean Purdy (a laboratory assistant), began experimenting with various forms of growth media, timing of implantation, embryo and zygote growth periods, and implantation techniques in the mid-1960s at Bourn Hall, near Cambridge, England. The next steps were to harvest sperm, as physicians had done for AI since the 1860s, and to fertilize the egg artificially. In order to streamline the process, Steptoe used laparoscopy—a noninvasive surgical technique that he first learned in 1958 from the French physician Raoul Palmer (1904–1985)—to gather sperm immediately from the vagina after intercourse. The laparoscope, first used for exploratory surgery, was more thorough and precise than the cannula for collecting sperm. The addition of a light source on the end of the laparoscope for better visibility was critical to the eventual success of IVF.[6]

Steptoe used the laparoscope for egg retrieval as well, as it could transport the eggs from the patient's reproductive tract to the laboratory safely. While "the laparoscope was a crucial technique for the move into clinical work," it took a steady hand to use it. The Australian physician John Leeton noted that it was especially challenging to use in cases of severe tubal disease or hidden ovaries, when patients had a so-called frozen pelvis (pelvic organs adhering together due to deeply infiltrating endometriosis). Steptoe and Leeton did not develop their own tools but used other existing surgical and laboratory tools to make egg retrieval and embryo transfer possible. These included a micromanipulator, an instrument for operating microneedles and micropipettes that the US-based scientist Ralph

Bannister first invented for cell surgery in 1912, and a microscope with a motion picture camera attached to observe the dissection of chromosomes.[7]

One further necessary technological step was the creation of a medium, or culture fluid, in which embryos could grow outside the uterus. A US-based researcher, Ralph L. Brinster (b. 1932), developed two different mediums in 1963 that could (1) support the development of mouse embryos to the eight-cell stage and (2) support the development of the eight-cell embryo to the blastocyst phrase. He also developed a technique that remains popular among IVF technicians and embryologists: "Brinster introduced cultur[ing] of eggs and embryos in small droplets of culture medium under a layer of paraffin oil. With some modifications, this 'micro-drop' method using the Petri dish has become the most widely used and successful system for culture of mammalian embryos in vitro." Though most present-day labs use mineral oil instead of paraffin, the technique and the Petri dish itself are still used in more than 95 percent of ART procedures.[8] The Cambridge team would adopt Brinster's technique and use of petri dishes; however, one of their colleagues would develop their team's own growth medium.

In Cambridge, the team "established a routine with two to three patients a month and tests with different culture media to try to cultivate five-day blastocysts, the point they thought optimal for introduction into the uterus." In 1968, one of their research associates, Barry D. Bavister (b. 1943), found a medium in which human embryos could survive that was based on one for hamster IVF. Two years later, he modified it to more closely resemble human follicular fluid.[9] However, those fertilized eggs did not survive long enough to be transferred into a patient's uterus. The role of a given medium in developing the "capacitation" of sperm—or their ability to transform physiologically and to penetrate and to fertilize the egg—is still poorly understood despite decades of experimentation and research.[10] Experiments with mediums and limited knowledge of capacitation hindered the Cambridge team's forward progress.

In Vitro Fertilization

Steptoe, Edwards, and Purdy were not the only researchers working on IVF. John Leeton and Carl Wood (1929–2011) led a different group at Monash University in Melbourne, Australia, and they achieved a short (less than one-week-long) IVF-generated pregnancy in a volunteer patient in 1973. However, the Leeton-Wood team's accomplishment was a singular event, and they did not repeat it until after the Cambridge team first used IVF on Lesley Brown (1947–2012).[11] Despite the Australian team's advances, Brown and the Cambridge team became famous overnight for making the first-IVF conceived live human birth possible. Brown received IVF treatment successfully using an egg generated from her natural cycle, and an eight-cell embryo fertilized with her husband's sperm was transferred into her uterus in November 1977.[12] In July 1978, that procedure resulted in the birth via planned caesarian section of her daughter Louise Joy Brown. Brown's birth was worldwide news and widely seen as a significant marker in reproductive technological history.

Following the announcement of Louise Brown's birth, many other medical teams tried to replicate the Steptoe-Edwards-Purdy model, to refine and to improve it, and to make technological breakthroughs of their own. The first IVF birth in Australia (and third in the world after India) took place in Melbourne in June 1980. The team at Monash University, which had been in contact with the Cambridge team since the late 1960s, had a series of successes with nine births later that year. Advances in new culture media, Leeton's expertise in laparoscopic egg collection, and "a new Teflon-lined aspiration needle that diminished turbulence and thereby minimized damage to the collecting eggs . . . together with a foot-operated suction pump for aspirating eggs from the ovarian follicles" all facilitated their achievement. The first IVF birth in the United States occurred in December 1981 in Norfolk, Virginia, under the supervision of retired husband-and-wife team Howard W. Jones (1910–2015) and Georgeanna

Seegar Jones (1912–2005), and a series of firsts in other countries followed.[13]

The potential of IVF quickly became obvious: it could bypass fertility problems such as damaged or blocked fallopian tubes, endometriosis, and poor sperm-mucus interaction and could help patients with these conditions achieve pregnancy. IVF had other effects in Roman Catholic countries: its success weakened doctors' adherence to prohibitions on masturbation for sperm donation and AI, and "accepting masturbation frees the path for IVF . . . to be practiced."[14] Physicians often placed a higher value on the (still only married) couple's desires for children than they did on religious strictures against masturbation and performed IVF on members of the faith. The ebb and flow of religious and legal restrictions—around who would do which procedure with whom and under what conditions—sparked the phenomenon of reproductive travel (chapter 4), in which would-be parents, physicians, egg providers, and for-profit companies move themselves and gametes around the world in order to make pregnancy and birth a reality for more people desiring children.

With the establishment of IVF as a standard procedure, new needs for medical technology and expertise in gynecologists' offices, fertility clinics, labs, and tissue storage facilities appeared. Each technique required investments in equipment, infrastructure, and highly trained staff. As Sandra González-Santos notes, "the introduction of high complexity ARTs meant a transformation of the gynecologist's workplace into an AR clinic, it meant the birth of the embryo lab, the emergence of the embryologist, the reconfiguration of the physician, the introduction of the administrative staff, and (more recently) the configuration of the AR nurse." Some gynecologists in Mexico, for example, who do not have the resources to operate independent full-service clinics, operate in a hub-and-spoke system in which groups of clinics outsource some elements of IVF (such as cryopreservation) to centralized facilities.[15]

Even if some elements are outsourced, establishing an IVF lab in the present is a significant investment. Labs need "high-tech equipment for conducting the procedures (such as micromanipulation systems, ovum aspiration pumps, CO_2 incubators, etc.) and environmental control systems and methods (such as special paint on the walls, double-filtered air, controlled temperature, controlled lighting, pressurizing modules [devices that maintain consistent air pressure], and laminar flow chambers [areas free of airborne contaminants])." The number of treatable patients, then, is limited to a clinic's infrastructural, technical, and human resources, as "the maximum number of patients they can manage per cycle depends on, for example, the number of incubators, nitrogen tanks, microscopes, and ICSI [intracytoplasmic sperm injection] benches they have, the number of embryologists on site, and the way these (humans and machines) work together."[16]

While the central activities of a fertility clinic's laboratory are the fertilization of eggs and storage of eggs, sperm, and embryos, many other tasks are necessary for them to occur and "to ensure the self-reproduction of the lab." Staff members stay busy with "the making of new culture media, the quality-control testing of the media on mouse embryos, the filling of the liquid nitrogen canisters for the freezers, and the ordering and receiving of new equipment and supplies."[17] Laboratory workers also need ongoing skill development to keep pace with technological development, and the equipment needs maintenance, repair, and periodic updating and replacement by yet another set of specialized technicians. The following sections examine how the IVF process has altered in the years since Louise Brown's birth through the mid-2010s.

As the outgrowth of IVF-adjacent technologies (aka add-ons or adjuncts) happens quickly, it is useful to take stock of the core process that has become more-or-less standardized in industrialized countries for the past twenty-five years. Sarah Franklin provided a snapshot of the process in the United Kingdom in 1997:

1.   previous infertility investigations to find source of obstacles

2.   choosing an IVF program

3.   initial work-up (including determination of ovarian reserve with measured serum levels of

follicle-stimulating hormone [FSH], measuring serum levels of anti-Müllerian hormone [AMH], and scanning the ovaries for a visual antral follicle count)

4.   preparation for first cycle, including drugs (one for ovarian activity suppression and daily or twice-daily doses of FSH using a syringe)[18]

5.   ovulation induction (daily drug injections, tablets, hormonal nasal spray, ultrasound scans, urine collection and sampling, blood tests)

6.   egg aspiration (human chorionic gonadotropin [hCG]) injection thirty-five hours before egg removal, valium/pethidine (pain medication) twelve hours beforehand, aspiration—surgical removal of up to thirty ova (general anesthetic may be needed), egg cultured with sperm in the lab

7.   embryo transfer (up to three through a fine embryo transfer catheter after twenty-four to forty-eight hours); patient must lie still for hours afterward[19]

8.   pregnancy testing after two-week waiting period

9.   prenatal monitoring if pregnancy has begun

10. birth, often premature and often by C-section.[20]

The likelihood of moving through these ten steps only once and ending with a live birth was dependent on a myriad of factors, including the genetic makeup of the couple's or donor's gametes, the would-be pregnant person's age and health, and the embryos chosen for implantation. A patient could also request that an egg is aspirated from a natural cycle instead of a super-ovulatory cycle, but the use of ovulation drugs is standardized in most practices (not to mention an additional source of clinic income). There are also medical risks that increase with age and certain health conditions, such as ovarian hyperstimulation syndrome (OHS), burst ovaries, ovarian cysts, migraines, and depression, especially if the procedures fail repeatedly. The process in 2015 in the United States, United Kingdom, and other countries with advanced technological infrastructures would often include preimplantation genetic screening (PGS/PGT-A) between steps 5 and 6 and ICSI between steps 6 and 7. Since the mid-2010s, even more optional "add-ons" are available, though some are accessible only to individuals with specific medical conditions (chapter 6).[21]

The IVF process has never been simple, but as more gynecologists, embryologists, and endocrinologists seek to improve the "take-home baby" rate in their clinics, more and more steps were added to the regularized process since Franklin outlined it in 1997. These additional steps, of course, take additional time and money and are not often covered by health insurance in the United States. There is also a psychological element at work: those who want a baby may feel that they need to include all of the extras, even if they are not medically necessary, to improve their chances of conceiving and bringing a pregnancy to term.[22] The following sections outline a range of IVF-related procedures, some of which have fallen out of favor, some of which have become standard in the recent past, and others that are becoming standardized in the present.

Gamete Intrafallopian Transfer (GIFT) and Zygote Intrafallopian Transfer (ZIFT)

Gamete intrafallopian transfer (GIFT) originated in San Antonio, Texas, in the early 1980s. An Argentinian-born, US-trained physician named Ricardo Asch designed a procedure in which eggs were removed as for IVF, but instead of external fertilization, sperm and egg were placed in the fallopian tube together. It was designed for couples who had fertility problems not located in the fallopian tubes and who had moral or religious objections to fertilization outside the body. The first live birth as a result of this process occurred in 1984, and Asch and his colleague Jose Balmaceda accepted an offer to move their practice to the University of California, Irvine. Eight years after Asch and Balmaceda moved, they and another colleague, Sergio Stone, were accused of financial fraud and misuse of eggs and embryos—

at least fifteen children were born from gametes that patients had not consented to donate to others. Asch and Balmaceda fled the United States to escape prosecution, and Stone temporarily lost his medical license.[23]

Despite this controversy, there were some minor advances in GIFT in the 1990s. While GIFT involved the insertion of sperm and eggs separately into the fallopian tubes to fertilize inside them, zygote fallopian transfer (ZIFT) involved the fertilization of an egg or eggs outside the womb. Then, that fertilized egg (zygote) was placed inside the tubes. In a comparable procedure called pronuclear stage tubal transfer (PROST), the zygote was transferred to the fallopian tubes at the pronuclear stage (after the sperm entered the ovum but before the genetic material of the sperm and egg fused).[24] However, the GIFT, ZIFT, and PROST processes are used only rarely in the present, given their complexity and lower rate of success as compared to IVF with ICSI. GIFT is part of fertility technology history not for advancing the field of fertility medicine, but rather as a warning that unscrupulous individuals have taken advantage of gamete donors in the past and could do so in the future.

Intracytoplasmic Sperm Injection (ICSI)

Intracytoplasmic sperm injection (ICSI), in which a single sperm is injected directly into an egg under a layer of oil, was first executed successfully in 1992. After IVF was standardized, research groups next investigated ways to help patients with low sperm count or azoospermia, and a team at the University Hospital of the Vrije Universiteit Brussel (Free University Brussels) in Belgium developed a technique called subzonal insemination (SUZI) on mice, which was "a micromanipulation technique involving the insertion of a few spermatozoa between the zona pellucida [outer layer of the ovum] and the membrane of the oocyte." The SUZI procedure was delicate, and occasionally one of the sperm entered into the cytoplasm of the oocyte. The researchers called this event "failed SUZI," but it was not a failure at all: after the sperm entered the cytoplasm, "we observed normal fertilization as well as embryo development . . . [and] called this procedure intracytoplasmic sperm injection (ICSI)." The first baby was born from this procedure on January 14, 1992, and "ICSI proved to be a consistent treatment for the alleviation of infertility due to severe semen abnormalities, including cryptozoospermia."[25]

To insert an individual sperm into an egg, it is necessary to master the microtools and related instruments, such as a large microscope with multiple controls, which make it possible for clinicians to follow their own actions closely. Five microtools are necessary: a holding pipette, a microneedle to create an opening in the egg, a biopsy micropipette, an angled micropipette, and a finely pulled micropipette for sperm insertion. As the tools need such fine calibration for each technician and the angle at which they operate, technicians sometimes like to make their own microtools using a microforge and beveler. Sarah Franklin describes their use in ICSI this way:

> The micro-tools are secured with small clamps that attach them to hydraulically-driven "joy sticks" that allow the manipulator to conduct various procedures, using touch as much as sight to guide his or her movements. The eyepieces are connected to a video lead that allows the manipulator to view the "bed" of the machine on a monitor, and to record, transmit, or display and further enlarge these processes on screen. To view the contents of a cell takes a practiced eye.[26]

Susan Martha Kahn, who observed these procedures in Israeli clinics in the 1990s, described how operators "slowed down the sperm in a chemical solution so that they could 'catch' one with microscopic tongs. They then manipulated the controls so that the sperm was inserted into the egg.... Once the egg had been penetrated with the pipette, [the lab technician] pressed a control that released the sperm and withdrew the pipette—a successful fertilization."[27]

In summary, the ICSI process allows "men previously considered infertile because of low sperm count or impaired motility to forego the use of a donor." If there are no severe sperm deficiencies, there is no major advantage to doing ICSI. Nonetheless, many individuals and couples opt to use it. One scholar identifies the advantages and disadvantages of using the procedure this way: "The excitement around ICSI has currently led to its overapplication, but it has also thereby put techniques developed for male body parts firmly into ART practice."[28] If anything, the procedure makes sperm-carriers more aware of the importance of their role in the IVF process.

Sex Selection, PGD, and PGT-A

Some tests used in conjunction with IVF raise questions regarding their association to eugenics. Ayo Wahlberg and Tine M. Gammeltoft refer to a distinction between assisted and selective reproduction as "the helping hand" versus "the guiding hand." Assisted reproduction, or "the helping hand," "aims to overcome biological obstacles to reproduction," while "the guiding hand," or selective reproduction, "aims to technologically prevent or promote the birth of certain kinds of children on the other."[29] Assisted reproduction includes procedures that help infertile individuals and couples become pregnant, but selective reproduction includes procedures that ensure children with or without specific traits are born. PGD and PGT-A tests are among the procedures that can be used for either assisted or selective reproduction, and their use is controversial.

Preimplantation genetic diagnosis (PGD), first conducted on humans in 1990, involves scanning embryos for genetic abnormalities, such as cystic fibrosis and muscular dystrophy.[30] Other types of preimplantation have not drawn quite as much debate. Preimplantation genetic screening (PGS), now known as PGT-A (preimplantation genetic testing for aneuploidy), began in 2007, and it involves scanning embryos for too many or too few chromosomes. PGT-A can indicate the presence of conditions such as Down syndrome and Turner syndrome, a condition that affects height and ovary development and causes heart defects in women. Spain is one country that does not restrict either of these tests. However, PGT-A "remains accessible only in private clinics where it is generally offered as an extra service enhancing the chances of success of the IVF cycle" and includes embryo biopsy. The problem is that "the biopsied cells . . . may not be representative of the embryo as a whole, leading to the risk of both false-positive . . . and false-negative results." PGD and PGT-A testing "contribute to the further blurring of a boundary that has always been blurred" regarding which children intending parents want to be born and which not.[31] A study published in November 2021 reporting data from fourteen Chinese academic fertility centers indicated that there was no improvement in the live take-home baby rate with PGT-A in the IVF cycles of 1212 healthy patients, casting further doubt on the relevance of the test.[32]

Egg Retrieval and Banking

Advancements in egg-retrieval techniques were ongoing in other research groups during Lesley Brown's pregnancy. In India, Dr. Subhas Mukerji used drugs to induce artificial ovulation and then froze the embryo before implanting it during his patient's next menstrual cycle. In October 1978, Kanupriya Agarwal was the second live IVF baby born and the first baby born from a hormonally induced cycle and an eight-celled cryopreserved embryo. Unfortunately, the Bengali Obstetrics and Gynecology Association rejected Mukerji's claim to success, and the West Bengal Government's Director of Health forbade him from publishing his work and mounting a defense of his achievement. Even though Mukerji was unable to claim credit for his work in his lifetime—he died by suicide in July 1981 and was not formally credited with the birth until 1997—his work demonstrated an alternate path to IVF success that future researchers could follow. The English researchers who facilitated Louise Brown's birth used natural cycles, hormonal dosage for ovulation timing, and high-tech laparoscopy for single-egg retrieval. Mukerji instead used a hormonally induced cycle, mucosal viscosity assessment for ovulation timing, colpotomy (transvaginal incision) for multiple egg retrieval, and cryopreservation of the embryos.[33]

In another area of research, the team at Monash University looked to increase the quantity of eggs as well as the quality. If more viable eggs were produced via artificial stimulation, they thought, the greater chance that one or more of those eggs would be usable for IVF. In 1981, they "introduce[d] hormonal stimulation cycles using human pituitary gonadotrophin (HPG) and clomiphene as a way to both increase the number of mature oocytes for harvest and control the timing of ovulation and oocyte collection." Embryos that were not implanted in one cycle could be frozen for later use in another, if needed. The production of more eggs than were needed for an initial round of IVF, combined with the technology to freeze the resulting embryos, facilitated the ability of patients to undergo additional rounds of IVF if the first one did not result in a successful pregnancy—or to request the implantation of more than one embryo per cycle. It also generated a host of moral, ethical, and legal problems regarding the patients' rights to use their own gametes, the risk of implanting more than one embryo at a time, the donation of gametes to others seeking children, and decisions about disposal if the tissues were not used. The gonadotropin-clomiphene treatment helped patients with fallopian tube problems but not those who produced nonviable eggs.[34]

In addition to using hormones to stimulate the production of multiple eggs, other physicians experimented with technologies beyond the laparoscope to gather them. One controversial and short-lived technique, known as uterine lavage or embryo flushing, involved eggs being fertilized in a donor's body and then "flushed" out for later insertion in the intending mother's body. The procedure never worked as intended—sometimes the embryo would not flush out, leaving the donor pregnant. Other donors developed pelvic infections or ectopic pregnancies or spontaneously aborted. The originators of the technique, the coincidentally named brothers Randolph W. and Richard G. Seed, thought that the technique would work in human women as well as it did in cattle. It did not.[35]

In a more successful experiment, a Danish doctor conducted the first transversal egg retrieval in 1981, with a needle through the bladder and general anesthesia with ultrasound guidance. Transvaginal retrieval was refined in France and Sweden in 1985, and a transvaginal ultrasound probe guiding egg retrieval was first used in 1986. In this procedure, the ultrasonographer sheaths the ultrasound probe in a sterile condom, coats the condom with jelly, and inserts the probe into the vagina. These "advances in ultrasound-guided egg retrieval transformed the first stage of IVF" and replaced the use of the laparoscope, which in turn reduced the need for general anesthetic to conduct egg retrieval. Laparoscopic surgery is still used as a diagnostic tool, now with monitors providing high-resolution, real-time images of the pelvic region so that the surgeon and assistants can see their instruments more clearly.[36]

Furthermore, IVF could be done with partial or complete donor gametes, and another series of firsts with donor gametes soon followed. The first successful pregnancy with a donor egg occurred in Melbourne in 1983 and in Thailand in 1987, and donor eggs for IVF first became available in the United States in 1987. By 1986, eight years after the first IVF baby appeared, the "take-home baby" rate in the United Kingdom was 9.9 percent, of which 24 percent were multiples.[37]

The retrieval of eggs, either for oneself or for someone else, remains a rigorous process in the present, with a pattern of steps similar to those done by the UK and Australian research teams starting in the 1970s. Retrieval occurs in an operating room, which contains anesthesiology tools, trays of instruments, cameras, screens, and bleeding control tools, among other standard equipment. "The injection of fertility medications stimulates the ripening of multiple eggs in the ovaries, a process that is monitored in physicians' offices through blood draws and ultrasound." Then, "when the eggs are mature, donors do a final 'trigger shot,' which causes the ovaries to release the eggs." Under ultrasound monitoring in the operating room, the physician guides a handheld instrument with a needle at one end into the follicle to take out the eggs.[38] If the eggs are to undergo fertilization immediately, they are transferred to a laboratory and prepared in a petri dish with culture media, many of which are now made with synthetic serum albumin (blood protein) instead of biological fluids. They are then fertilized via ICSI or placed in a petri dish with washed sperm for approximately eight hours while fertilization ideally occurs.

Even though both egg and sperm donation involve the removal and retrieval of gametes in one body to combine with those of another externally, the world of egg donation differs starkly from the world of sperm donation. Artificial insemination, as we have seen, became a regular gynecological procedure in many countries in the last quarter of the nineteenth century, and sperm banks had existed since the 1950s. Egg banks began to appear in the United States only in the late 1980s, as oocytes did not survive cryopreservation with glycerol the same way that sperm did. Scientists eventually found another medium, propanediol (which can be derived from glycerol), that cryopreserved eggs relatively well, though some also used dimethyl sulfoxide (DMSO). Oocyte preservation would advance significantly with the advent of the Cryotop, a storage mechanism (see below).[39]

Along with this development in cryopreservation media for oocytes, the establishment of egg banks as commercial enterprises began in the 1990s and coincided with the development of the Internet. It is no wonder that egg and sperm banks around the world turned to the Internet to advertise their gametes directly to interested recipients and to find providers (a term now more commonly used than "donors"). As a clinic's website is its first point of contact with potential providers, it must be carefully structured to stir positive emotions by emphasizing the benefits of provision and deemphasizing its downsides. On some Spanish egg provision websites, for example, "egg donation is portrayed as aligned with progressive moral values, female empowerment and social justice." Clinic websites pair these loftier sentiments with reassurances about the normalcy of egg donation in young women's lives, together with "the promotion of fun through consumerism and the promotion of self-care and agency."[40] In this framework, egg provision is a progressive act demonstrating self-determination that in turn can inspire other women to do the same.

The need to channel the interests of potential providers toward altruism combined with the pleasures that compensation and subsequent consumption can buy is also true of fertility companies that offer clients provider eggs and surrogacy together. In that arrangement, egg providers travel to the surrogate's or intended mother's location to facilitate IVF and implantation without cryopreservation as an intermediate step. Potential egg providers must be convinced that the benefits of travel—perhaps framed as a vacation with other providers who could become friends—outweigh the physical unpleasantness and potential health risks of the provision itself: "The circulation of hope is found throughout the mediated donor narratives, combined with the orchestration of fun. In these narratives, the discomforts of travel, medication injections, and the uncertainties of medical procedures in a foreign place is turned into a fun tourist experience."[41]

One example of this kind of cross-border egg provision takes place in South Africa, which has become a hub for global egg agencies over the past decade. After an egg provider got ovarian hyperstimulation syndrome overseas in 2009 (she recovered), the South African Society for Reproductive Medicine and Gynecological Endoscopy (SASREG) banned local agencies from making overseas trips. However, international agencies based in South Africa are not regulated by SASREG and are not subject to the ban. Egg providers in the late 2010s through the present tend to be Afrikaans—white women often from poor rural areas seeking opportunities to earn money and to travel to countries including Cyprus, Cambodia, the United States, India, Ghana, and Nepal. As Amrita Pande observes, "this biolabor is built on young women's aspirations for cosmopolitanism." They also accept less payment for eggs than white women in the United States—their average compensation per cycle is US $2,000, compared with anywhere from US$4,000 to US$15,000 per cycle in the United States.[42] However, surrogates are rarely included in these visions of paid holidays and fun, and their work lasts much longer than that of the donors.

The role of payment in gamete provision structures the experiences of egg providers; "no other human tissue is so systematically ordered through significant money transactions." Though egg donation is an involved and time-consuming process, and eggs are sold at a high price, many agencies shun women who state financial instead of philanthropic motivations. At one US agency, "Women who attempt to make a 'career' of selling eggs provoke[d] disgust among staff, in part because they violate the altruistic framing of donation."[43] The many steps between egg provision and birth distance donors from recipients, which serve a dual gendered purpose: providers distance themselves from the retrieval process and potential future children so that they are not subject to personal feelings or outside accusations of being bad mothers (a good mother, the thinking goes, would care for any child born of her genetic material), and intending parents separate IVF and implantation from provision so that they feel like genuine mothers (where femininity = fertility). These are hard psychological needles to thread for all involved.

Eggs are particularly difficult to preserve, as they are the largest cells in the human body.

Cryopreservation and Vitrification

Whether someone is undertaking egg extraction for themselves or someone else, the retrieved eggs undergo another process if they are not used right away: cryopreservation. Improved cryofreezing techniques made egg and embryo freezing possible from the early 1970s onward. "Egg freezing, or oocyte cryopreservation," Lucy van de Wiel writes, "is effectively an IVF procedure with a prolonged period of cryostorage after the eggs' extraction from the body, but before their fertilization. While the eggs are in the freezer, stored at –196 degrees C in liquid nitrogen tanks, they are thought to be unaffected by the passage of time." Eggs are particularly difficult to preserve, as they are the largest cells in the human body (0.1 mm in diameter) and have a large liquid volume sensitive to ice crystal formation.[44]

The process of vitrification has improved the process of cryopreservation of eggs in particular: "To vitrify is to transform a substance into 'glass,' to render it stable and inert through very rapid cooling to about –100°C, at which point molecular activity ceases. . . . Flash freezing, combined with appropriate cryoprotectant, generally preserves the tissue structure by lowering the freezing point and reducing the time taken to move from fresh to frozen state." The vitrified eggs "do not so much exist *in vitro* (in glass), but rather are *vitreum* (as glass) within the liquid nitrogen tanks." The means of egg storage—both during vitrification and thawing when ready for use—was critical to the establishment of vitrification as a technique: the Cryotop, a storage device developed in Japan in the early 2000s, "proved pivotal in raising the eggs' post-thaw survival rates up to 90%."[45] Oocyte vitrification was declared no longer experimental by the European Society of Human Reproduction and Embryology (ESHRE) in 2012 and by the American Society for Reproductive Medicine (ASRM) in 2013, allowing companies like the Kitazato Corporation to enter the vitrification business.[46]

The Cryotop is a thin strip of transparent film attached to a liquid nitrogen–resistant plastic handle. It comes in different sizes and can store up to four oocytes per device in its internal straw. It is sold alongside a range of accessories necessary to operate it, including equilibrium and vitrification solutions, a Repro Plate (for performing freezing and thawing procedures), a Cooling Rack (to contain the liquid nitrogen), Aluminum Blocks (to hold the Cryotops steady during insertion and sealing), a Heat Sealer (to seal the straw in which the oocytes are stored shut), and a Straw Cutter (to cut the straw when the oocytes are ready for use). A video of the cooling procedure shows a technician piping a small amount of the equilibrium solution and vitrification solution into the Repro Plate's wells, equilibrating the embryo or blastocyst (exposing it briefly to a low dose of cryoprotectants that shield it from damage), transferring it to the well with the equilibrium solution, removing it from that well and swirling it briefly around the two wells with vitrification solution in a pipette, aspirating the excess solution, transferring it with a minimal amount of solution to the Cryotop, plunging the Cryotop into the liquid nitrogen, and finally covering the device's inner straw with an outer straw and capping it while keeping it submerged in the liquid nitrogen.[47] The process takes steady hands and patience to manage, not to mention a close eye on the tissue under the microscope. Though few clinic patients may see the Cryotop, its accessories, the laboratories, the laboratory technicians, or the storage facilities in which the Cryotops are stored, the existence of these devices, people, and sites affects the actions and thoughts of patients, egg donors, and clinics regarding egg freezing specifically and fertility generally.

Cryopreservation rearranges reproductive time in three different ways for patients, egg donors, and clinics. First, for patients, "the capacity to cryopreserve women's fertility is having decisive effects on the overall shape of the oocyte economy, creating new forms of exchange, distribution, and value." It affects how clients think about the age at which they would most like a child and their ability to plan the timing of a pregnancy as precisely as the gametes and their bodies will allow.[48] Cryobanks encourage young people to freeze their own eggs in order to preserve them for pregnancy in later life. Patients with a medical diagnosis, such as BRCA mutations (tumor-suppressing gene mutations that are prevalent among Ashkenazi Jewish women), cancer, or any condition with treatments that may lead to sterilization, often have medical insurance that covers the procedure. For patients without a diagnosis, it is called "private," "social," or "elective" egg freezing, and medical insurance—even in pronatalist countries like Israel—rarely covers it. In 2019, elective egg freezing costs approximately £3,755–£4,728 in London, $4,000–$7,000 in Israel, and $10,000–$15,000 in the United States, with additional yearly storage fees of $500–$1,500. Women may seek out these services themselves, or private companies may offer them to employees.[49] As Jenna Healey argues, "the reconfiguration of biological time is not just a by-product of the modern life sciences, but also a significant source of capital for the biotechnology industry."[50]

Given the availability of voluntary egg freezing in the United States and United Kingdom, among other highly industrialized countries, reproductive aging and timing is now an aspect of health that egg-carriers with uteri can anticipate, monitor, and manage. Egg freezing is just one among several practices now known as "fertility extension technology," which "shifts the boundaries of reproduction, as well as normative conceptions of infertility, by extending the period of time in which women can realize motherhood." In other words, women and other egg-carriers can anticipate infertility and can invest in services that (probably) will help them avoid childlessness in the future. If they do not make those investments, the implicit logic goes, they have only themselves to blame.[51]

Second, in cases where a donor provides a fresh egg, the process has to be coordinated carefully with the recipient. Donation can be anonymous, or the donor and recipient could potentially know about each other. In either case, the process can feel intimate on both sides, and the clinic has a role in managing the emotional as well as the physical and financial sides of the transaction. "Fresh donor cycles are highly personified transactions, even when they are anonymous. . . . The egg bank is simultaneously a legal, commercial, and technical facility."[52] Donors and recipients alike may see fertility counselors for support during the transaction.

Third, for clinics, "the ability to freeze and thaw reproductive tissues dramatically increases clinical traction over synchronization and the husbandry of reproductive potential."[53] Cryopreservation and vitrification, in other words, are not only storage technologies but sophisticated means of tissue organization and management. Frozen eggs and other reproductive tissues become part of technological infrastructures managed by networks of for-profit corporations. So, the decision to freeze eggs is not simply a decision to guard against potential future egg declination or infertility. It is a decision to enter into a long-term economic relationship with a company that will inevitably shift over time due to the client's personal circumstances, the company's stability, or new scientific findings. In other words, "egg freezing . . . becomes an entry point into a long-term, technologically managed reproductive trajectory across the life course."[54]

If clinics manage provider eggs as well as eggs from women who freeze eggs for their own use, they may solicit egg providers from the surrounding area; others use an additional set of technologies to transport gametes from one part of the world to another. Transport technologies can deliver gametes from donors to recipients or to surrogates. As Catherine Waldby notes, "the history of cryobiology is the history of preservation *and* transportation." The banking of human tissues requires cold chain security, and international regulations and cold chain infrastructures shape how eggs and other tissues are moved within countries and internationally. Logistics companies like Cryoport specialize in the transport of semen, embryos, and other reproductive tissues around the world: "They use dry vapor dewars [cryogenic storage containers], liquid nitrogen, insulation transport, tracking technology, chain of custody documentation, and an entire suite of logistics to ensure the preservation of fertility across space."[55] Clinics and logistics companies must work together to navigate regulatory regimes and technological requirements to ensure the safe transport of tissues across hundreds or thousands of miles.

The decision to freeze eggs is not simply a decision to guard against potential future egg declination or infertility but to enter into a long-term economic relationship with a company.

Specialized preservation technologies and logistics planning, all under the careful eyes of professionals, make these movements of gametes across geographies and national borders a reality. They also depend on combinations of new technologies with long-standing ones, such as airplanes (in which nitrogen vapor preserves the tissue) and trucks (in which nitrogen liquid preserves the tissue). With the development of cryopreservation in the second half of the twentieth century and vitrification in the mid-2000s, "each reproductive segment can be realized in different places," and thus reproduction "has become transbiological, transtemporal and transnational in hitherto unimagined ways while introducing possibilities of selection at each step."[56]

How successful is IVF? It depends on who you ask, how they define success, how they keep statistics, and whether those statistics are publicly available through the clinic itself, a governmental agency, or a professional, accrediting organization. Not all countries or professional bodies require fertility clinics to submit their statistics or to publish them, nor do they all conduct audits of clinics. Data submission and analytic parameters vary from country to country and from organization to organization. Data sets usually include the number of eggs fertilized in IVF, the number of blastocysts transferred (and whether they were single or multiples), the number of IVF cycles that led to pregnancies, the number of caesarian sections, and the number of preterm deliveries. More fine-grained statistics include the usage of ICSI, PGS, or PGT-A; indicate whether the gametes were from the patients or donors; and state whether the gametes were fresh or frozen. Most potential clients of a clinic are interested in the "take-home baby" rate, or the percentage of clients who take home a live child (or multiples) at the end of treatment, and those statistics help individuals and couples determine if a specific clinic is right for them.

In a review of results from Australia and New Zealand in 2012, the live delivery rate per IVF cycle for all women was around 14–17 percent. In a 2014 report from the National Center for Chronic Disease Prevention and Health Promotion, 40.5 percent of all US women under thirty-five years old had a live birth after treatment, but only 1.8 percent of women over forty-four did. The UK's Human Fertilisation and Embryology Authority publishes an annual statistical report compiled from clinics countrywide. The 2021 report on 2019 data stated a live birth rate of 32 percent per embryo transfer for patients under thirty-five years old and below 5 percent for patients who were forty-three years old or older. At the same time, the percentage of patients seeking IVF treatment at the age of forty or older increased from 10 percent in 1991 to 21 percent.[57]

These correlations between success rate and age and the number of patients over forty years old seeking treatment also held true in Central and South America. The Latin American Network of Assisted Reproduction (REDLARA), an organization that certifies IVF centers in fifteen countries, compiled statistics for its nearly 200 member clinics in 2018. The REDLARA report stated that the number of procedures is growing fastest among women forty years or older, and 32 percent of treatments were for that age group. The take-home baby rate (aka the delivery rate) for all age groups was 18.5 percent with ICSI and 19 percent with IVF alone.[58] From this brief overview of statistics in different parts of the world, it is clear that the success of IVF is dependent on a myriad of factors, of which age is only one among many.[59] However, if the number of older patients seeking IVF continues to grow, researchers may turn increasingly to improving their treatment odds.

As Naomi Pfeffer puts it, "fertilization in vitro and embryo transfer represent the first innovations in the treatment of infertility developed by a gynaecologist since Rubin introduced the tubal insufflation test shortly after the First World War."[60] These processes were indeed the first major innovations in the field since the 1910s, but many smaller innovations and discoveries in earlier decades set the foundation for IVF to become a success. In summary, "the emergence of IVF can be analyzed as a continuous but dialectical history of biotechnical innovation that derives from deliberate human intentions, and response to specific desires and hopes, while simultaneously transforming the terms through which new aspirations are imagined."[61] IVF and its successor technologies have dramatically shifted the parameters of fertility diagnosis and reproductive treatments in ways that Rubin never could have imagined. These technologies have ramifications across national legal structures and for religious believers, and their use has altered patterns of reproductive travel as gamete providers and seekers pursue and find each other. The next chapter examines some of the legal, religious, and travel-related effects of IVF around the world.

LAW, TRAVEL, AND RELIGION

With each development in assisted reproductive technologies, national regulatory bodies, public and private insurance companies, for-profit companies, and religious authorities decide how to structure access to and use of them. However, not everyone seeking a child agrees with their local regulations or religious directives, and they travel to other countries for services that they cannot access locally—or arrange for a gamete provider to come to them. As Amrita Pande and Tessa Moll write, "geopolitical factors that shape circuits of resources, patients, and technologies include non-availability of technology and procedures at home, legal restrictions on certain demographic groups, high costs, and long waiting lists for procedures."[1] National differences in ART regulations, including the age at which one can undergo fertility treatment, anonymity (or lack thereof) for sperm and egg donation, and the use of surrogates lead to reproductive travel for service-seekers and egg providers.

While some efforts have been made to make IVF and its accompanying procedures available to lower-income individuals in under-resourced countries, existing patterns of reproductive travel illustrate how law, religion, finances, and personal decision-making perpetuate existing economic inequalities in the global fertility industry. Motivated individuals and couples with financial means can circumvent legal limits by traveling to countries where limits are less strict or nonexistent, creating "reproductive pathways" or "reproflows" for "reproductive travelers." Further, "such reproflows exist within a larger 'reproscape,' or a complex, transnational, reproductive health landscape characterized by circulating peoples, technologies, body parts, media, finance, and ideas."[2] Those "reproflows" also change over time according to shifts in national legal and regulatory frameworks, as is clear in the cases of Romania and India outlined below. Egg and sperm banks, egg providers, surrogates, and those seeking gametes (not to mention the gametes themselves) move around the world in different patterns according to market forces, sometimes skirting the law.

Law

Great variation exists among countries regarding limits on access to fertility technologies and procedures based on age, health, sexual identity, marital status, or other traits. Laws, policies, and regulations are often created in response to scientific developments and do not anticipate them. In other words, "the rapid rate at which reproductive technologies unfold means they often leave in their trail a complex web of legal, ethical, social, and regulatory questions which the government has no option but to address, often in haste and trying to catch up with a fait accompli."[3] The following examples are only three among many possible angles into fertility technology regulation: how under- or overregulation affects providers' and child-seekers' experiences, restrictions on certain services requiring decision-making on a case-by-case basis, and disputes over the use of stored gametes.

First, countries where assisted reproductive technologies are lightly regulated or unregulated can be uncertain terrain for those seeking pregnancy. To take one example, in Lebanon, "there is no local IVF scientific registry of any sort . . . thus, there are no reliable statistics on the numbers of IVF cycles with and without donation." Furthermore, "'fresh' sperm samples are used in sperm donation, without any kind of mandatory screening," and "no mandatory genetic testing is performed." Lebanon is also the only Muslim-majority country aside from Iran that permits egg donation, paving a "reproductive pathway" there for egg donors and potential clients. The absence of legislation or regulation may be due to a lack of resources, a national interest in producing Lebanese citizens, and/or a professional medical interest in maintaining a market for profitable fertility services. Put colloquially, "Lebanon has now taken the former place of Italy as the 'Wild West' of Mediterranean fertility treatment."[4]

On the other end of regulatory oversight, Romanian authorities decided to enforce strict rules on egg provision and sales after staff at an Israeli firm, Global ART, were accused of exploiting egg providers for their own profit. Following the Global ART case, Romanian authorities established a ban on commercialized or paid ova provision (Law 95/2006 Regarding the Reform in the Health System), so that only voluntary and exclusively altruistic egg provision was legal. Anyone involved in an egg-centered financial transaction, from the child-seeker to the egg provider to the fertility clinic staff, could be prosecuted as a trafficker of gametes.[5]

Under Law 95/2006, it became much more difficult to find local egg providers for the transfer of fresh eggs, unless they were close relatives of the child-seeker. Gamete banks were also illegal, so anyone seeking pregnancy via IVF had to find a genuinely altruistic provider, pay a provider illegally, or purchase foreign gametes from fertility clinics. At the same time, "a national programme aimed at helping IVF patients tackle infertility was set up in 2011 and, with a 3-year break between 2012 and 2015, it has been financed up to this day [2018]. State support consists in one free cycle of IVF for heterosexual couples using their own gametes."[6] Law 95/2006 obviously clashes with federal programs that promote fertility, so the gamete regulatory situation is at a stalemate. And where Romania was formerly a country providing eggs to Israel, it now imports them, often from Spain—changing the direction of its reproflows.

Second, some treatments are available only on a case-by-case basis in some countries, such as preimplantation genetic diagnosis (PGD) in conjunction with human leukocyte antigen (HLA) tissue typing. That procedure "enables parents who already have a child affected by a fatally genetic disorder to have another baby whose stem cells, taken from the umbilical cord, can 'cure' the existing child, a so-called 'savior sibling.'" The rights of parents to move forward with the process are subject to approval by national regulatory bodies or nonpolitical advisory committees appointed by them, not individual physicians. These include the National Commission of Human Assisted Reproduction (Spain), the Human Fertilisation and Embryology Authority (United Kingdom), and the Advisory Committee on Assisted Reproductive Technology (New Zealand).[7] These committees are responsible for reviewing individual requests to use this technology and then issuing rulings on them.

The main ethical concerns related to this procedure are whether coming into existence to save a sibling psychologically harms the children created to do so, and whether the use of ARTs for these situations "is unethical or contrary to public morality." In other words, the use of this procedure is acceptable if the older child's life is threatened without the existence of the new sibling, but not if the older child has a more minor, non-fatal illness. A 2000 case in the United States (for an older child with Fanconi anemia, a bone marrow disorder) and two 2001 cases in the United Kingdom (one for an older child with beta thalassemia, a genetic blood cell-production disorder and another for Diamond-Blackfan anemia, a sporadic blood condition) brought the ethical debate into public view. In the United States, the request was approved, and in the United Kingdom, the first family was approved to use the procedure and the second was denied, a decision that was later reversed. Nearly two decades later, the US case of Molly Nash and her savior sibling Adam is a success, and Adam still feels responsibility for his sister but was not psychologically harmed. PGD testing continues to be regulated closely, so that children are not born to donate any body part beyond blood or bone marrow for their older siblings or to donate to any person except a sibling.[8]

Third, as cryopreservation of sperm, eggs, and embryos can keep genetic material viable for many years, there are ethical concerns with the storage, disposal, and future research use of these materials. As part of a position-paper series on ethics in the mid-2000s, the European Society of Human Reproduction and Embryology (ESHRE) recommended that adults should have moral and legal autonomy over the fate of their gametes and that clinics should make the client's wishes regarding their gametes' future legally binding. Four options exist: the gametes can be destroyed; they can be used for research and laboratory training (sometimes but not always at the same clinic); the clients can pay for storage; or the gametes can be donated to other individuals or couples seeking pregnancy. However, clinics do not always enforce their own rules. A physician interviewed for the *New York Times* in 2019 stated that clinics do not always discard embryos, even if a client has stopped paying storage fees, as they are nervous that a client may return and sue them for destruction of tissue anyway. While the United Kingdom has a maximum fifty-five-year cap on cryopreservation of embryos, the United States has no cap, and so that physician's concern could become reality.[9]

Other ethical and often religious problems arise if, for example, a couple divorces but one person wants to use the genetic material; if one spouse dies, the other wants to use the genetic material, but the family of the deceased objects; if a couple stops paying for preservation of their frozen embryos; or whether a private company or publicly held cryopreservation bank adheres (or not) to religious criteria regarding the disposal of, or research on, embryos. If the clinic operates in a conservative Christian framework, its owners, staff, and clients may view embryos as "persons" or "pre-born children" already imbued with human rights, making the physically simple process of discarding tissue a major moral problem. Some clinics offer clients the opportunity to dispose of their unused embryos in a religious ceremony and bury them formally. Over the past decade in the United States, "embryo adoption" services that match unused embryos with couples who want them for IVF have opened around the country, but they restrict the matching process to married, Christian, and heterosexual couples. Of course, not everyone shares that moral framework and thinks that embryo distribution should be restricted that way. As one recent international study of clinic discard practices put it, "the undefined moral status of the human embryo remains to be one of the most significant ethical dilemmas that has surfaced in the world of assisted reproduction technology."[10] It is not likely to be resolved anytime soon.

Minimal regulation in Lebanon, overregulation in Romania, PGD with HLA tissue typing restrictions, and the management of discarded gametes are only some examples of the many ways that laws and regulations, interpretations thereof, and the extent to which these laws are enforced structures the use of ARTs. These laws, practices, and regulations vary widely around the world, and access to different services and body products have led to patterns of international reproductive travel, or reproflows.

The next section examines some of them and the reasons why they exist.

Travel and Access

Many fertility and preimplantation technologies (outside home-based AI and timing methods) are dependent on highly skilled technicians and infrastructure and are time-consuming and expensive if not covered by health insurance. There is a persistent inequality of access to specialized fertility technologies, as some are available only to those with the money, time, and health to pursue them: "economic stratification not only shapes people's access to technology but also determines how they are positioned in relation to it."[11] In turn, people in less-resourced countries are often the providers of gametes or surrogacy to people in wealthier countries. To take one example, as egg donation in Denmark is allowed but poorly compensated, the country has a "double role as a fertility hub in the production of donated sperm (and its use) and its role as a producer of fertility travelers in search of both eggs and embryos." As of 2018, if travelers find sperm but not eggs, they can obtain eggs from elsewhere (often Spain) to combine with Danish sperm and then return to Denmark to receive IVF. Sperm sales are only lightly regulated, so anyone outside the country who is interested in Danish sperm can either travel to Denmark for artificial insemination or have cryopreserved straws shipped to them. As intrauterine insemination and IVF have been allowed for lesbians and single heterosexual women as of 2007 (and for any woman up to age forty-six), older, lesbian, and single heterosexual female travelers can look to Denmark for fertility services.[12]

To take another example, the fact that egg donation is also illegal in Germany and Switzerland (and was until 2015 in Austria) has spurred citizens of those countries to travel to Hungary, the Czech Republic, or Spain for donor eggs. The ban on donor eggs in Germany is enforced under the 1991 Embryo Protection Act (*Embryonenschutzgesetz*), which forbids elective single embryo transfer, surrogate motherhood, and egg donation on the grounds that a child needs to know its mother. Medical border crossing and health tourism from Austria to Hungary is common, and reproductive travel is part of that larger pattern. Although egg donation is allowed in Hungary, very few eggs are available, because providers (as in Romania) cannot be paid—but illegal payment sometimes happens behind the scenes. Native Hungarians who have moved away also return to their home country if they need donor sperm or eggs, in the hopes of having children who have a similar heritage.[13] As egg freezing technology continues to improve and become more widely available, "frozen egg trajectories are developing along existing pathways between wealthy nations with egg shortages and popular donor-egg IVF destinations with relatively permissive egg-procurement regulations."[14]

Potential reproductive travelers seeking donor sperm, eggs, or embryos for themselves must take both legal and financial factors into account when contemplating traveling overseas for fertility treatment. Italy's restrictive Law 40/2004, "Norms on the Matter of Medically Assisted Procreation," forbade artificial insemination by donor until it was partially overturned in 2014, so Italian individuals and couples seeking donor sperm in the interim needed to find it elsewhere. From 2007 to 2011, a sociologist regularly interviewed a single Italian woman in her forties, "Linda," who first explored becoming pregnant via the less-expensive option of AI with donor sperm, which had a low success rate compared to IVF. She looked into IVF at a Belgian clinic, but the 5,000-euro cost deterred her. After some more exploration, she chose a 1,500-euro IVF procedure at a clinic in the Czech Republic, which offered to implant embryos that others had relinquished during their previous treatments.[15]

A different kind of reproductive pathway exists in West Africa, where medical training in IVF is not available — specialists must fly in to perform the technique—and the two clinics in the region that offer IVF are both in Accra, Ghana. As their clinic directors are "to a large extent free to decide how they perform assisted reproductive technologies," the two clinics structure their patient care around the long distances that patients must travel, often from countries such as Gabon, Nigeria, Ivory Coast, and Burkina Faso. In the Lister Clinic, women were encouraged to remain in the hospital for five days after the embryo transfer procedure, and in the Pro Vita Hospital, women were required to stay until they could take a pregnancy test. If they tested positive, it was strongly recommended that they remain hospitalized until the pregnancy could be confirmed by fetal ultrasound, usually two to three more weeks. Doctors in both clinics used the same basic reasoning to justify these recommendations—Ghana's bad road conditions and the high cost of IVF. Most couples paid for treatment themselves, and hospitalization increased clinic income. They heard about the clinics through word of mouth and did not ask about success rates. While "the seemingly high level of transnational reproductive mobility across West African borders may reflect the high overall transnational mobility in the region, mainly for commercial reasons," IVF services are nevertheless rare in West Africa.[16]

Surrogacy is yet another form of reproflow that has shifted directions over the last decade. Its practice comes with legal, financial, and medical hurdles for all participants involved, even those with the best intentions. Misuses and abuses of surrogates have become public knowledge in the past decade, with India and Thailand as prominent examples of where these problems have taken place. The Baby Gammy case in the latter country magnified the problems of commercial surrogacy and drew international attention. In 2013, an Australian couple hired a Thai surrogate, Pattaramon Janbua, who became pregnant with boy-girl twins. An ultrasound at four months found that the boy had Down syndrome and a heart condition. The couple asked her to abort the boy, but she refused. After birth, the couple took the girl back to Australia and left Gammy with Pattaramon. The scandal over the couple's decision to abandon their disabled child—compounded by the revelation that the father was a convicted sex offender—led to legal reform. Thailand banned commercial surrogacy and restricted it "to heterosexual couples married for at least two years, at least one of whom must be Thai, and surrogates must be relatives."[17]

Surrogacy in India was also the target of reform around the same time. India began permitting surrogacy agencies to operate in 2002, and for thirteen years, it was a hub for individuals living in countries where surrogacy was prohibited who sought surrogates for their own or donated gametes. However, due to poor living conditions, inadequate medical care, and low payment for surrogates, the federal government banned international commercial surrogacy in August 2015. The ban shifted the focus of Indian reproduction-oriented businesses from surrogacy to embryo fertilization and exportation thereof to countries that have not restricted surrogacy. As Amrita Pande points out, "India is now a grey zone of pre-conception assemblage—a hub where eggs and sperms are assembled into embryos, frozen and/or exported for gestation in women in countries with no surrogacy regulations." Indeed, "the only effect of the ban has been to push the surrogacy industry elsewhere, increase gestational mothers' precarity and absolve the government from paying attention to critical questions around globalization, reproductive justice and international law."[18] Based on public activism and outcry, legal protections can be strengthened against potential human rights violations of surrogates and the children they bear; however, risks remain in countries where surrogates have inadequate legal protections.

Given the uneven availability of sperm, eggs, and IVF treatment facilities, alongside inequalities in income, health insurance, government regulations, and medical facilities, travel for reproductive purposes will continue to increase. Reproductive travelers of various ages, health concerns, sexual identities, and marital statuses will travel to different countries to obtain genetic material and reproductive medical care or to provide gametes. Their gametes may travel internationally with their consent but beyond their ability to control who receives them. Absent international regulations regarding the age at which one can receive fertility treatment or hire someone for surrogacy (among other potential barriers), reproductive travel will continue to shift from one country to another.[19]

Religion

Religion and ethics play a distinct role in determining the use or nonuse of specific fertility technologies and procedures. As Gayle Davis and Tracey Loughran point out, "medical and moral discourses" are "impossible to separate . . . medical belief and behavior have been bound by potent social codes and used to enforce social norms."[20] These morals and ethics are particularly visible when it comes to examining religious responses to, and guidance on, the use of assisted reproductive technologies. World religions have different theological reasonings for permitting or banning AI, IVF, or other ARTs. This section outlines the perspectives on IVF put forward by Roman Catholicism, Sunni and Shia Islam, and Judaism. Their similarities and differences are based on each religion's understanding of how marriage functions as the institution within which human life begins.

Roman Catholicism

Beginning with a pronouncement on March 26, 1897, that artificial insemination was illicit, Pope Leo XIII

(1810–1903) and his successors as heads of the Roman Catholic Church have forbidden all artificial methods of promoting birth as interference with the marital act between husband and wife. Pope Pius XI (1857–1939) proclaimed the encyclical *Casti connubii* (On Christian Marriage) in December 1930, which forbade contraception and adultery (in cases where the wife was sterile, and the husband wanted children) and addressed artificial insemination indirectly. The text emphasized that sexual intercourse within marriage was "the means of transmitting life, thus making the parents the ministers, as it were, of the Divine Omnipotence." Pope Pius XII (1876–1958) issued three further pronouncements in September 1949 (to a congress of Catholic doctors), in October 1951 (to a gathering of Catholic midwives), and before the Second World Congress on Fertility and Sterility in May 1956 in Naples, Italy. The 1956 statement was clear and to the point: "Artificial insemination is not within the rights acquired by a couple by virtue of the marriage contract, nor is the right to its use derived from the right to offspring as a primary objective of matrimony."[21]

Thirty years later, Cardinal Joseph Ratzinger (b. 1927), later Pope Benedict XVI, released *Donum vitae* (Instruction on Respect for Human Life in Its Origin) in 1987, which condemned the use of all ARTs for the Church's followers. Artificial insemination, even in the context of marriage, is forbidden, as it robs the act of sexual intercourse from its value as a means of conception and marital union: "Fertilization achieved outside the bodies of the couple remains by this very fact deprived of the meanings and the values which are expressed in the language of the body and in the union of human persons." Indeed, no technology or physician can replace "the specific act of the conjugal love of [a child's] parents," as it is the act itself that both connects the married couple and "transmit[s] life to a new person."[22] Single women or widows are also forbidden from becoming pregnant via IVF, as is IVF with a surrogate for any believer.

The only licit means of creating human life, in the Church's view, is through penile-vaginal intercourse between a husband and wife and subsequent emission inside her vagina. Any other means involves masturbation and third-party objects, and thus interferes with the unitive and procreative purpose of sex. In other words, "a life that is created by medical practitioners—rather than through an act of conjugal love between two married people—'establishes the domination of technology over the origin and destiny of the human person.'" The use of donated gametes also has an association with infidelity, as it does in Sunni Islam. The Church does permit surgical intervention to remove obstructions due to endometriosis and ovarian wedge resections (partial removal of an ovary), which remove internal blockages due to polycystic ovary syndrome (PCOS).[23] These surgeries are allowed because they do not interfere with heterosexual intercourse.

Assisted reproductive technologies make families in a wide range of configurations possible, and they can subvert the traditional vision of heterosexual, cisgendered, and two-parent families central to Church theology. However, ARTs can sustain and perpetuate the gender norms that the Church promotes as well. For example, as the prohibition against masturbation for extracorporeal sperm production for IVF was increasingly ignored in Mexico in the 1990s, literature and media about the topic increasingly emphasized IVF as a means to uphold Catholic ideals of devoted motherhood following the model of the Virgin Mary: "Because it is Marianistic mothers [that] the Mexican AR system is producing, assisted reproduction acquired force and was deemed acceptable." If the Virgin Mary is the ultimate example of womanhood and motherhood, true "women should sacrifice everything they have for their children (or children to be) and [should believe] that science—aided by God—is capable of everything. Assisted reproduction strengthens one more very important element in the Mexican construction of motherhood, the element of sacrifice."[24] In this case, the relative importance of one religious stricture was deemphasized (regulations against male masturbation) and another was emphasized (women's adherence to ideals of Marian motherhood). Within a rigid theological framework, some Mexican Roman Catholics have found a way to use ARTs that nonetheless affirms their commitment to the faith.

Fernando Zegers-Hochschild, a founder and chair of REDLARA, sees the role of religion in decisions about AI and IVF in a different way. "Many people in Latin America argue that IVF has taken procreation out of the hands of God. It is my belief that this revolution is not an attempt against those who believe that children result from God's will; on the contrary . . . having children for many women results only if thorough and technologically sound work is undertaken with the help of science."[25] It is impossible to know how many ART users in the past or present are Roman Catholic, and the extent to which they know or take this teaching to heart. Through the promulgation of *Donum vitae*, the Roman Catholic Church places the tightest restrictions on the use of ARTs for its followers of any worldwide religious organization.

Sunni and Shia Islam

In Sunni Islam, IVF has been allowed only for married couples using their own gametes since 1997, and the freezing of embryos created with a husband and wife's gametes is permitted. When IVF was becoming established in the United Arab Emirates, non-Muslim couples could provide donor gametes in UAE clinics. In 2010, though, the UAE passed a federal law declaring strict new regulations for clinic use. Freezing embryos, among other practices allowed for Sunni Muslims, was now forbidden. As mentioned earlier, Sunni Muslims who want to pursue IVF now travel to Lebanon, even if their coreligionist physicians in their home countries would not agree with their decision. "Although most Sunni IVF doctors and patients remain firmly against such practices, Lebanon has become a hub for 'reproductive tourism,' primarily of Sunni Muslims from other Middle Eastern countries where donor gametes and technologies are unavailable."[26]

Shia Muslims in Iran can use donor technologies after a fatwa (nonbinding but authoritative religious proclamation) from Ayatollah Ali Hussein Khamenei in 1999. Egg donation is allowed for Shia Muslims under the teaching of "temporary marriage," in which a sperm or egg donor can become a legitimate but temporary spouse, so that the donation is within the bounds of legal marriage. Embryo donation and surrogacy were also legally approved on the same grounds in 2003, if the embryo donation comes from a married couple and is given as a gift to the child-seeking couple. In addition, Shia scholars make a distinction between natural seminal fluid and specially prepared sperm for assisted reproductive technology. The latter "technosemen" is more acceptable, as it distances the donor from the recipient through the technological processes of washing and centrifuging. Sunni authorities consider artificial insemination with donor sperm syringed into the vagina as adultery or fornication (*zina*), while most Shia authorities argue that the word *zina* must be restricted to "penile penetration of the vagina" and therefore donor insemination with prepared sperm is not classifiable as *zina* and thus allowable.[27]

Judaism

The association of fertility and gender manifests in another way in contemporary Judaism. Jewish perspectives on IVF and related technologies are intertwined with historical and more recent Jewish theology, along with the history of Israel as a modern state. The state encourages all Jewish women to have children to maintain the population of believers and has established policies to make IVF available to any Jewish woman who wants it. The state has procedures for sperm donation that reflect its prioritization of generating Jewish children: to wit, "the specific identity and origin of sperm is conceptualized as irrelevant to Jewish reproduction."[28] Relatedly, Jewish theology has had to address the religious implications of IVF generally and for unmarried or divorced Jewish women and their family structures specifically. These religious perspectives have a range of consequences as well, including forbidding Palestinians in prison from accessing ARTs.

Israel has one of the most generous state-supported AI and IVF programs in the world. Every Israeli woman under forty-five years old is eligible for unlimited free rounds of IVF treatment up to the birth of two live children, and women aged forty-five to fifty-four are entitled to unlimited state-subsidized egg donation. If selected for AI or IVF, the patient receives anonymous sperm donations from donors chosen by social workers in one of twenty-five clinics. The social workers take the recipient's preferences into account—most often, the recipients want sperm from donors who were also Jewish and resembled them—but make the final selection of donor themselves. This process is somewhere in between the free market donor choice in the United States and the lack of donor choice in China (chapter 2). In Israel, "unmarried women's consent suggests that they do not imagine themselves as 'consumers' who are entitled to pick and choose goods in the reproductive marketplace, as has been observed in other contexts," writes Susan Martha Kahn. "They understand their pursuit of conception as part of a more communal process of reproduction."[29]

As "Israeli Jewish women are left as the primary agents through which the nation can be reproduced as Jewish," whether or not women are married is less important from a population growth perspective. On the one hand, unmarried Israeli women face some additional challenges, such as finding a *mohel* (circumciser) who will perform circumcision for a male child with no father listed on his birth certificate. On the other, state-supported IVF provides lesbians who do not want a sexual relationship with a man the opportunity to become mothers. The primacy of motherhood for all women, regardless of sexual orientation or marital status, "remains understood as a deeply natural desire and goal, despite the extraordinary technological measures necessary to achieve it. The cultural importance of motherhood thus becomes reinforced through unmarried women's use of reproductive technology at the same time that the meaning of motherhood has become transformed."[30]

The Aloni Commission Report on the Matter of In-Vitro Fertilization in 1994 brought together state and religious viewpoints on IVF into a single document. The Report supported an unmarried woman's right to access IVF "as part of her basic right to privacy." As a result of this commission, the rights of Jewish women to access IVF are protected under both religious and secular law, and "the rabbinic pragmatism vis-à-vis the new reproductive technologies works to reinforce the Halakhic imperative to be fruitful and multiply."[31] Not only was a woman's right to access services protected in this report, but state and religious authorities also established regulatory control over IVF clinics.

IVF clinics in Israel have rabbinical observers on staff, who oversee the practices of physicians and other staff members to ensure that they uphold Halakah (the Jewish oral laws that supplement the scriptural law), especially around menstruation. Clinic staff have translated Halakhic ideas about purity and impurity into clinical and surgical protocol. For example, a clinic doctor "performs an oocyte pick-up in such a way as to avoid rendering the woman a *niddah* [one who is ritually unclean] as a result of the procedure." The observers and staff know each other well, and they develop a collaborative work community around their respective duties. IVF clinic work, like much other work in medicine, "has also become routinized in the workplace and . . . the people who work to achieve conception have come to see their tasks as entirely ordinary."[32]

These services are not available to everyone, though. The ongoing conflict between Israel and Palestine impacts the ability of Palestinians to access fertility services and the gametes of men in prison for AI or IVF. As Gala Rexer writes,

> If a person with a Jerusalem ID is married to a West Bank resident and they want to have children by using ART, bodies and body parts have to literally cross borders: a sperm sample has to traverse the checkpoint controlling and surveilling Palestinians' movement and access to Israel, frozen and parceled, or the West Bank partner has to cross the border him- or herself to receive treatment in an Israeli hospital.

For Palestinian political prisoners who wish to have children with their partners, this problem is especially acute. Since 2012, prisoners, their wives and families, NGOs, and fertility clinics practice "biopolitical resistance: they manage to smuggle a sperm sample of the imprisoned husband out of the Israeli prison and into a fertility clinic in the West Bank or Gaza." Thus, prisoners' sperm travels across borders from the prison, across the Green Line that separates Israel from the Occupied Palestinian Territories, and then into the fertility clinic where AI takes place, and Palestinians are not always welcomed, to say the least.[33] The efforts of Palestinian prisoners, their families, and NGOs show clearly that religion and politics shape access to reproductive health care and services and that people will go to extraordinary lengths to make their hopes of pregnancy a reality. Restricting access to fertility services and the pursuit of pregnancy are both political acts.

In sum, religious teaching regarding what is permitted and what is forbidden continues to evolve, and religious strictures can intersect with politics and national and international laws. Laws and religions shape reproflows and reproductive travel, whether that travel is by whole persons or by gametes transported by others. As Sarah Ferber and colleagues note, "changing regulatory regimes have produced a checkerboard of subnational, national, and international laws and regulations that have, in the context of increased fertility travel by providers and clients, generated a transnational momentum that regularly switches and redirects the clinical practice of AR."[34]

Reproductive travelers seek services outside their home countries for any number of reasons and circumstances, including age, gender, sexual orientation, citizenship status,

Restricting access to fertility services and the pursuit of pregnancy are both political acts.

availability of certain services, and finances. The examples described above illustrate the extent to which people sacrifice money and health and risk arrest in pursuit of pregnancy—and that some, such as egg donors and surrogates, may also risk their health to provide services to others. ARTs are clearly not neutral technologies. Their use takes place within wider contexts that illustrate relationships of power between individuals, religious authorities, political regimes, and the law.

TECHNOLOGY, KINSHIP, AND FAMILY

Fertility technologies generally and assisted reproductive technologies in particular shift the meanings of parenthood, kinship, and family. The availability and use of ARTs in a country have long-term political and financial implications as well, especially regarding government investment in population growth. As Sandra P. González-Santos observes, "ARTs are not simply technologies that help people have children . . . they can be political tools to prove how modern and technologically advanced is a region, a country, a health system, or a local medical group; they can also be 'a technology of social contract,' a way of responding to the sociocultural values assigned to kinship, gender identity, and lineage."[1] This chapter explores these issues and the multiple ways that individuals, identity groups, clinics, and countries have managed their approaches to ARTs. It examines how race and imaginings of race are incorporated into donor gamete selection. It studies selective reproduction for disease avoidance and gender selection, the role of gender in the ART process and feminist critiques thereof, the challenges of queer individuals and couples in accessing ARTs and forming kinship bonds, and, finally, the emotional and financial toll that ART processes can take on those engaging with them. Given the ever-expanding complexities and add-on treatments involved, seeking a child not only involves significant health risks, but also the risk that they may not work at all.

Racial Concerns

Racial issues in ARTs include how clinics recruit donors; how clinics identify and classify the race of sperm and egg donors; how prospective parents categorize their own racial identity, especially as it relates to the prospective racial identity of future children; and how IVF-born children (especially those with different racial and ethnic backgrounds than their parents) understand and come to terms with their own racial identity. This section focuses on the second and third of these issues—it begins with how race classification for donated sperm began in the 1980s, then moves to how race manifests in embryo donation organizations, the production and valuation of whiteness and a reflection on the broader meaning of race in ARTs, and finally shifts to selective reproductive technology.

Race as an element of choice in AI began with the catalogs that nonprofit sperm banks first produced in the early 1980s. These banks catered to lesbians desiring anonymous sperm donation, so that they could self-inseminate and raise children without the biological father's knowledge or involvement. Catalogs included basic phenotypical information about donors, such as eye color, hair color, and height. As a staff member at the Feminist Women's Health Center in Oakland, California, observed in a newsletter:

> Most sperm bank donors are blond-haired, blue eyed—Aryan. So what happens with the mixed couple that is infertile? They have no place to go. We are going to have such a wide range that women will really have a choice. The information which will be entered in the donor catalog will include height, weight, race, hair color and texture, eye color, sexual preferences, the occupation of each donor and educational background.

Long before for-profit banks took over sperm donation, the absence of racial variety among donors was an issue. And after the AIDS crisis led many nonprofit banks to close and for-profit banks with cryopreservation and testing facilities to open, "the idea of a consumer choosing the hereditary qualities of a donor . . . became taken up . . . by a new generation of commercial sperm banks."[2] Race became a component of gamete choice in banks early on, with the phenotype of volunteers or paid donors not aligning with client interests serving as a point of frustration.

More recently, the centrality of race in egg and embryo donation has become visible in non- and for-profit agencies, including US-based Christian organizations started in the 2010s that redirect unused and unwanted embryos from disposal or scientific experimentation by offering them to infertile couples. The anthropologist Risa Cromer observed that clinic staff try to match embryos with intending parents based on how alike they and the providers look—along with their racial background as stated in written applications: "While the application presents race as a self-evident object, the everyday work of classifying donors can produce race as a contingent, unstable, and sometimes conflicting set of 'relations established between a variety of entities.'" Cromer highlights the consumer-centered nature of this process, illustrating that "responding to client desires for resemblance in gamete donation and transnational adoption has had commodifying effects in which prospective clients come to behave like shoppers for ideally racialized 'products.'"[3] By attempting to match embryos with intending parents based on appearance, agencies use physical likeness as a proxy for genetic relationship in an attempt to satisfy clients' wishes.

Some intended parents prioritize "whiteness" of gametes over other characteristics. To take one example, donor whiteness sometimes manifests as the idealization of a Nordic body type and coloring. At one Danish clinic in the 2000s, advertisements for donors showed how "skin colour is reworked as a matter of choice, and it primarily serves to facilitate commercial communication among white consumers." The whitening of gamete donors in Ecuador in the early 2000s involved clinics deliberately recruiting lighter-skinned egg and sperm donors. In general, they tried to match the skin color of the patients seeking gametes, but if there was not a close match, "practitioners would pick a donor lighter than the recipient." One clinic staff member said explicitly that the director did not want indigenous donors because "he wanted to 'mejorar la raza' (better the race) through mixing."[4] That desire for whiteness structures some clinic's approaches to seeking providers.

A frequent client preference for whiteness is clear in the case of South African egg providers. As mentioned in chapter 4, egg providers with Afrikaans backgrounds have a high value on the global gamete market, as their genetic material produces a form of whiteness in children that passes as Northern European whiteness at a lower cost than white US egg providers demand. "The kind of whiteness purported in South Africa and claimed as a boon to its international draw in the fertility market, is lacking in ethnicity, geographical specificity, and professes a globality that is unreachable to other white locales. . . . Matchers [at fertility agencies] use the similar settler colonial history as a selling point."[5] Taken together, these examples from Denmark, Ecuador, and South Africa of the value of white gametes show how providers, agencies, and intending parents can agree on means to manifest whiteness in future potential offspring.[6]

This "traveling whiteness" also manifests in the imaginations of intending parents who do not identify as white, but who want one half of a child's genetics to be from a white gamete provider. Amrita Pande calls these imaginings "strategic hybridization," the existence of which illustrates how "racial imaginaries and notions of race and whiteness are manipulated, transformed and put to new use." Some couples desire a form of "mixed whiteness" for their potential children, which has become "a marker of desirable otherness in terms of esthetics—mixed race *white* individuals are celebrated as embodying beauty, cosmopolitanisms, and metrosexuality." This form of mixed-race whiteness "does not challenge racial hierarchies" but instead "is a specific kind of mix that will allow the next generation to access their parents' privileges (in terms of class privileges) but also be technologically enhanced through a strategic hybridization of the local familiar and the 'top race.'"[7]

Intending parents wanting a child that looks like them—a desire that appears uncontroversial at first glance—is deeply problematic.

Examining race in ARTs shows how deeply some child-seekers value whiteness in their potential future offspring and the desires of intending parents to have children who resemble them—often at a very high price. In addition to following patterns of economic inequalities, "global ART markets tend to reproduce racial hierarchies, as they are prone to benefit people who have higher social status and exploit those who do not."[8] Meanwhile, those who want gametes from providers of color have a more difficult time finding them. More broadly, it shows how much control some intending parents want to exert over a highly technical process, and how the values of individual choice in consumer capitalism extend to the manifestation of a specific desired child. As Camisha A. Russell reflects, ARTs "reinforce existing inequalities in local and global labor markets . . . [and] reinforce the privileging of whiteness and the naturalization of racial categories."[9] In short, intending parents wanting a child that looks like them—a desire that appears uncontroversial at first glance—is deeply problematic, as it not only reinforces racial hierarchies, but also gives rise to unrealistic expectations that a potential child will not just look like the intending parents but *be* like them.

In another vein of embryo selection regarding a potential child's health, the process of selective reproduction (in the form of preimplantation genetic diagnosis [PGD] and preimplantation genetic screening [PGS/PGT-A]) influences the type of embryos that physicians and users seek to implant. Clinics conduct PGT-A tests to detect chromosome translocation, which is a possibility when women have several miscarriages or implantation failures and want the "healthiest" embryo possible implanted. They can also be used when women know their hereditary disease status and want to avoid passing diseases onto their future children. Fertility clinic staff use the test results to advise would-be parents regarding which embryos to implant. Reading the embryos is still more of an art than a science, and in these cases, there is not a clear boundary between assisted reproductive technologies and selective reproductive technologies.

A commercial technique derived from PGT-A is MicroSort, which enables clinicians to separate out sperm with X and Y chromosomes. Couples can then avoid having children of one sex if they have a hereditary history of a sex-specific disease. MicroSort uses ICSI to insert the gendered sperm into the egg before IVF. The company and fertility clinics often refer to spermatic selection with IVF as "family balancing," but it can obviously be used in patriarchal societies to avoid having girls. However, the company's argument is that the application of this technology "could avoid abortion by establishing desired pregnancies based on characteristics in the resulting child."[10] Even if true, that reasoning does not address the sexism underlying a decision-making framework in which prospective parents would abort female fetuses simply because of their gender.

Selective reproduction is currently available to avoid neurodegenerative and hypertrophic myocardial pathologies, for example. However, it is not available to select for specific traits, such as those related to appearance—a manifestation of the "helping hand" versus "guiding hand" distinction described in chapter 3. The fact that prospective parents could someday make "designer babies"—and eliminate any trait that they may consider a "disability"—is a distant but vivid possibility. Taking racial preferences and health concerns together, it is clear that "IVF is undergoing a new change, from a solution to involuntary infertility to a novel form of optimisation via utilising and capitalising on whiteness along with racialised imaginaries and desirabilities."[11]

Fertility and Reproductive Justice

ARTs are open to criticism not only regarding their ability to reify racism and embryo sex selection. Criticisms of ARTs from a feminist perspective began not long after the birth of Louise Brown. In the early 1980s, second-wave feminist scholars and journalists identified ARTs on a continuum of technologies that a patriarchal medical hierarchy used to control and to manipulate women's bodies.

Most prominent among them in the United States were Janice Raymond (b. 1943) and Gena Corea (b. 1946), and Corea's 1985 book *The Mother Machine* exemplified that perspective. For them, reproductive technologies were akin to genital mutilation, coerced pregnancy, forced sterilization, and sex-selective abortion or infanticide—any practice or procedure that valued men's desires and preferences over women's control over their bodies. In short, reproductive technologies were "transforming the experience of motherhood and placing it under the control of men."[12]

Two of Corea's main criticisms of ARTs were male physicians' control over technological development and use and the medical community's indifference to the pain that women endured during ART testing and treatment. After outlining the development of tissue and embryo freezing in cattle and its application to human women, she notes that "medicine is not just a healing art but an institution of social control. IVF gives the power structure [doctors] potent tools for such control." She also noted the absence of pain in the triumphalist narratives of Louise Brown's birth, highlighting passages from Lesley Brown's memoir that illustrated the bleeding and pain Lesley endured throughout the IVF testing process, particularly after laparoscopies.[13] Corea did not provide a solution to the problems that she identified, but rather called on women to be aware of the potential harms of further intrusions of reproductive technology in their lives. Though women are no longer compared to cattle, and the number of female physicians has grown markedly since the book was published, her point that women's physical and emotional pain is underacknowledged in reproductive health care remains trenchant in the present.

This kind of wide-sweeping feminist evaluation of ARTs has rarely been heard since. To take one example of more current commentary, in 2009 Jennifer Parks reflected on Corea's and Raymond's work and raised no objections to ARTs per se, but rather called on feminists to encourage its use in the formation of queer families, not heteronormative, patriarchal families. "If they are going to persist," she argues, "we should ensure that women who are marginalized by their skin color, sexuality, ability status, marital status, and age are not denied access to the technology. . . . I am not arguing for a rise in the use of ART, but in the proportional use by marginalized groups."[14] Criticism of ARTs in the more recent past focuses not on whether feminists should reject these technologies wholly—that is now a moot point—but rather on identifying ways that ART access, use, and gamete provision can be accessible, fair, and equitable for all. As ARTs become ever more deeply embedded in the international reproductive landscape, it becomes more important to address equity in access internationally to be sure that everyone in the industry is paid and treated fairly and is free from abuse or neglect in their medical treatment. Forbidding them from reproductive health care would not stop the practice of ARTs but likely drive it underground.

Queer Families and Reproductive Justice

A framework for identifying and redressing inequity in fertility technology access, use, and provision is reproductive justice. As ARTs "have the capacity to effect deep social, cultural, ethical, biological, and ontological changes," the study of fertility technology will increasingly view decision-making, policies, research and development, distribution, legalities, and use through the lens of reproductive justice. Reproductive justice positions the availability of contraception, fertility technologies, and environments for child-rearing in a broader context of women's rights and human rights, based on the United Nations' Declaration of Human Rights and Article 16, which includes "the right to marry and to found a family," and the statement that "the family is the natural and fundamental group unit of society and is entitled to protection by society and the State." Just who can be named as a family and who has these specific rights is a central question for the administration of law and justice around fertility. Although "certain sorts of impediments to founding a family are unlawful," and an individual's procreative decisions are a human right, that right

Just who can be named as a family and who has these specific rights is a central question for the administration of law and justice around fertility.

has limits: it "does not entitle one to positive assistance in founding a family" in all countries across the world.[15] However, some countries, including Argentina and Uruguay, do include universal access to assisted reproduction as part of a citizen's reproductive rights.[16]

The Declaration of Human Rights, even though it does not guarantee access to fertility services to all global citizens, is nonetheless a source of inspiration for theorists and activists. A prominent example is the way that US feminists of color have used the Declaration of Human Rights as a foundation for their thinking and advocacy on reproduction. They first outlined reproductive justice in the 1990s and codified it in the early 2000s. One common definition from Asian Communities for Reproductive Justice (now Forward Together), written in 2005, is as follows:

> Reproductive justice is a movement-building and organizing framework that identifies how reproductive oppression is the result of the intersection of multiple oppressions and is inherently connected to the struggle for social justice and human rights. Reproductive justice argues that social institutions, the environment, economics, and culture affect each woman's reproductive life.[17]

A reproductive justice perspective provides a lens for identifying how certain groups of people are allowed or disallowed access to fertility technologies on account of personal characteristics, most often marital status, sexual orientation, citizenship, and financial status. Reproductive justice has three umbrella principles: "(1) the right *not* to have a child; (2) the right to *have* a child; and (3) the right to *parent* children in safe and healthy environments." These principles illustrate "the need for protection from coerced sex and reproduction and also from coerced suppression or termination of fertility." They are especially important as a guiding framework for action when fighting for the rights of disadvantaged groups, and the second principle is most critical to equity in the use of, and access to, fertility technologies. "Although single people, same-sex couples, and especially trans people once faced enormous obstacles in getting access to reproductive technologies, once technologies are made available, people will find a way to access them—despite the obstacles."[18] Though there are still indeed obstacles, there is plenty of resistance to them.

One example of attempts to restrict access to ARTs is in Indiana, when in October 2005 the state legislature tried unsuccessfully to pass a law that would have made any AI users other than heterosexual married couples guilty of "unlawful reproduction." Another is in Denmark, where acquiring donor sperm was forbidden to lesbians and single women from 1997 to 2006. To challenge that regulation, a lesbian midwife named Nina Stork found an intermediary to buy sperm and used AI to inseminate clients, and as a result of her advocacy, Danish lesbians and single women could receive AI beginning in 2007. An example of loosening restrictions occurred at the end of June 2021, when the French parliament passed a bill that allowed lesbians and single heterosexual women to access IVF, permitted elective egg freezing, and gave children conceived with donor sperm the right to know the identity of the donor when they become adults. France was the eleventh of the twenty-seven European Union nations to allow same-sex IVF.[19] Taken together under the second reproductive justice principle—the right to have a child—it is possible to measure the effects of legal actions on reproductive rights. A reproductive justice perspective illuminates inequalities in access to technologies across national boundaries and cultures and provides a framework for action to remedy them.

Reproductive justice is not limited to heterosexuals but is instead inclusive of all persons who aim to have children or to limit their fertility freely and autonomously. The use of AI and ARTs by gay, lesbian, bisexual, transgender, and non-binary individuals is sometimes similar to and sometimes different from their use by single and coupled heterosexuals. Recent interviews with fifty-one Anglophone men, trans/masculine, and non-binary persons who sought ART services showed that they decline donor requests for conception via sexual intercourse and reject the idea that conception must be difficult for them. They may be less likely to concern themselves with physical resemblance to their children and more likely to develop a kin relationship with their sperm donors, developing their own constellations of family and kinship beyond heterosexual, two-parent, nuclear family norms.

Families in which the sperm donor is part of a child's extended family but not the child's day-to-day life are creative in naming their relationships. For example, one set of parents calls their sperm donor "spuncle" and his parents "grandspuncle" and "grandsparkle."[20] For non-binary individuals, "cisnormativity and heteronormativity influence each stage of non-binary people's journeys. . . . assumptions that people's body parts, gametes, gender, sex, sexual orientation, and family configurations are all inextricably linked underpins these normative ideologies."[21] Transgender, queer, and non-binary individuals manifest conceptions of family and kinship on their own terms, and those terms may or may not align with ideals of cis- and heteronormative families. What all users or potential users of ARTs have in common, though, are the aging, health, and cost issues that come with their use.

Financial and Emotional Concerns

ARTs can take a toll on the bodies, finances, and romantic relationships of those who pursue them. News and media

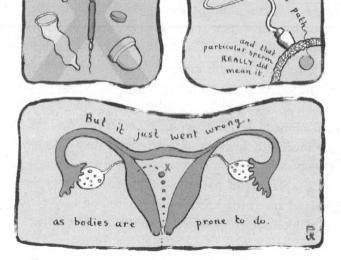

Figure 8 Paula Knight, "It Was Never Meant to Be," 2012. *Source:* Courtesy of the artist.

about women giving birth past menopause, gestating their own grandchildren if their daughters cannot carry a fetus to term, or birthing high numbers of multiples (such as Nadya Suleman, aka "Octomom") gives many people hope that they too can have "miracle babies."[22] It is challenging to weigh the risks and benefits of proceeding with ARTs with the physical, financial, and emotional factors at play, especially if the procedure continues not to manifest in a desired pregnancy. A comparative study of IVF costs in the mid-2000s in different countries states the average cost per live birth as $41,132 in the United States, $40,364 in the United Kingdom, $24,485 in the Nordic countries, and $24,329 in Japan. Those without personal savings, private insurance, or the assistance of public health insurance may accrue significant debt at a high interest rate to finance ARTs. In 2006, Capital One Fertility, a division of Capital One Finance Corporation, offered loans of up to $40,000 to child-seekers at interest rates up to 25.99 percent.[23] As the costs of high-technology fertility treatments continue to rise, and the number of possible add-ons grows, individuals and couples must decide for themselves how much money, time, and energy they can invest in ARTs.

A 2021 study of patient decision-making regarding add-ons in the United Kingdom centered on the role of hope in determining whether or not to use them. The authors found that some patients make cost-benefit analyses before agreeing to add-ons, some accept all add-ons despite the cost, and some see unproven add-ons largely as ways for private clinics to make money and are skeptical of them. One patient described their approach to deciding this way:

> The fact that you're already paying ten grand [£10,000], it doesn't matter, you know, and you'll do anything and you know, the whole thing is a bit of scientific experiment . . . it's sort of not blind faith but your hope is such that you, if someone says something will work then you might tend to go for it. . . . You're just paying a lot of money for hope and . . . the add-on *is that*, isn't it?

Even if patients had the financial means to include all of the add-ons they wanted, however, decision-making had an emotional cost. Some patients "expressed a sense of being burdened by the responsibility of navigating the treatment options that are available to them. . . . Evaluating add-ons is thus connected to patients' broader acknowledgement of the many unknowns and uncertainties associated with IVF."[24] As add-ons are constantly under development and have unproven track records, and for-profit clinics are motivated to make money as well as to help patients, patients make complex and costly medical decisions without neutral advice.

Access to and advances in fertility technology are linked to broader shifts in public and global health practices related to contraception, sexual health, pregnancy and abortion care, and sexually transmitted infection prevention and management (including HIV/AIDS prevention and management). The ability of clinics to obtain the supplies that they need to perform IVF, to hire and train staff, and to gain certification from national or international standards boards is a constant need, especially in under-resourced countries. Any changes in national or international laws regarding gamete donation, transport, and surrogacy; the policies and practices of nonprofit or for-profit clinics; and the manufacturing practices, cost, and distribution of medical supplies all impact the worldwide availability of IVF. That availability translates into the ability of individuals and couples to seek and to use reproductive health services. It also impacts people's imaginings of what their families could look like—whom their children could be—and how they could establish networks of kin and family with the assistance of technology.

Individual and societal concepts of kinship and family will continue to alter given the multiple manifestations thereof that ARTs permit. These concepts will not only change within families and among parents, but also in citizenship rights and other kinds of legal rights. And if technologies are available only to people who can afford them—if states allow fecundity only for their wealthiest citizens—there are eugenic implications regarding the abilities and rights of all citizens to reproduce. Fertility technologies are embedded in some of the deepest human questions about founding a family, the human-technological relationship, and the meaning of kinship. In other words, "reproductive technologies make our assumptions about the workings of kinship, biology, and gender explicit."[25]

FUTURE DIRECTIONS

As new developments in ARTs are happening all the time, there will be corresponding scholarly and political attention to global feminist organizing around sex and reproduction, including the right to fertility through technological means. However, the future of fertility technology is not only in ARTs. Different points along the path toward pregnancy attract diverse innovators with creative approaches to fertility problems. Technologies with historical longevity will undoubtedly stay in use. This chapter begins with innovations in sperm manipulation and diagnostics, moves to the ways that people use historic technology with modern touches, and then considers advances in the technologies related to IVF, known as adjuncts or add-ons. It concludes with an overview of uterine transplant technology and the possibility of conception beyond gender. There is no shortage of academic, for-profit, nonprofit, medical, and potential client interest in tackling fertility problems and improving the success rate of fertility technologies across the globe.

Semen and Technosemen

The health of sperm remains an important area of diagnostic concern. Low sperm count, low motility, irregular morphology, varicoceles (enlarged veins in the scrotum), damaged sperm ducts, hormonal deficiencies, testicular failure, and sperm antibodies (proteins that damage or kill sperm) are all sources of infertility. Sperm health is difficult to treat, and some workarounds for those with at least some healthy sperm include testicular sperm extraction (TESE) and testicular sperm aspiration (TESA), which involve "special high-powered needles and delicate microsurgical instruments [to] take sperm directly from the testicles." Physicians can also do testicular mapping, a process of "fine needle aspiration (FNA) used to see what areas of the testes, if any, are producing sperm."[1]

In addition to technologies that can help manifest pregnancy, the gametes themselves can be thought of as technologies. This is true of technosemen, or semen that has undergone laboratory manipulation to be suited especially for ICSI and IVF. Matthew Schmidt and Lisa Jean Moore define it as "the 'new and improved' bodily product

Gametes themselves
can be thought of as
technologies.

that semen banks advertise to clients. . . . Technosemen is the result of technologically based semen analysis and manipulation." These manipulation methods include the swim-up method, which means "centrifuging the semen sample, removing the seminal fluid, and placing the remaining sperm pellet in an artificial insemination medium. After an hour, the most motile and active semen which 'swim' to the top of the solution are retained." Another method is Percoll washing, which involves layering the semen with a cleansing solution and centrifuging it for half an hour.[2]

The ability to manipulate and to choose the best semen affects how clinics view their donors, their donations, and the children who might result from them. For example, in advertising materials for the Danish company Cryos, "semen is solely described in light of the technology involved. . . . traces of the matter are reworked into sophisticated technology, beautiful children and indeed—and not surprisingly—happy, healthy, potent donors." This view that semen is a technoscientific product, not a body product, likewise manifests in China in two ways: first, the country's Ministry of Health established specific requirements for technosemen under national law from 2001 to 2003. The Ministry requires a concentration standard of 60 million sperm cells per milliliter, which is "four times higher than the World Health Organization's criteria for normal male fertility." A range of "technologies of assurance" quantify spermatic quality not only according to sperm per milliliter, but also "motility grades, percentages of normal morphology, and milligrams of fructose per milliliter."[3] Then, only the best sperm is used to make the "best quality" children.

Second, the ability to test spermatic health is a means of managing the effects of environmental pollution on the next generation. In cities like Wuhan, semen donated on days with high levels of air pollution showed lower sperm count and concentration than semen donated on days with lower levels of air pollution.[4] The processes of fertility medicine that remove other kinds of impurities are necessary to counter the negative effects of pollution. Washed technosemen is perceived as healthier and more potent than natural, unmanipulated semen. Sperm banks can then "make claims about the potency of their products, while at the same time making claims as to the 'naturalness' of new reproductive technologies. These constructions suggest that new reproductive technologies are not unnatural but rather an improvement upon the inherent unpredictability of natural procreation." In other words, "the best semen is not natural; it is processed and refined through technology."[5] The technologies that produce "technosemen" counter others, like environmental pollution.

Diagnostics

Some of the technologies and procedures first established in the early twentieth century for fertility diagnosis remain a part of the medical landscape, including laparoscopy (for diagnosis, if not for egg retrieval). Most prominently among these is the hysterosalpingogram, the X-ray procedure used to determine blockages in the fallopian tubes. As the functionality of the fallopian tubes often needs investigation as well, physicians can conduct fluid ultrasonography (FUS) with a sterile saline solution using a vaginal ultrasound; a tuboscopy, in which a thin telescope is passed through the fimbriae (fringed edges) of the fallopian tubes to evaluate their inner structure; and a falloscopy, in which a fiberoptic tube is guided through the cervix and uterus and into the fallopian tubes. Other diagnostic possibilities include a selective hysterosalpingogram, in which a thin, flexible catheter is run inside a hysterosalpingogram (HSG) catheter that can also clear tubal blockages. One additional set of measurements is tubal perfusion pressure (TPP) measurements. If the tubes are too rigid or diseased, they "may not be able to sweep the released egg into the tubal opening, thereby making an eventual conception impossible."[6]

The hysterosalpingogram, like some other diagnostic and treatment technologies, is also adaptable to circumstances in which the full range of IVF technologies is not accessible. The Belgian obstetrician/gynecologist Willem Ombelet has spent much of his career developing IVF services in Ghana, and he points out that "since tubal obstruction associated with previous pelvic infections is the most important cause of infertility in many African countries, hysterosalpingography and/or hysteron-salpingo-contrast-sonography are affordable techniques to detect this problem." In addition, he advocates the use of a mini-hysteroscopy to investigate intrauterine abnormalities, a procedure that "has been simplified in its instrumentation and technique, so that it can become a non-expensive diagnostic technique for every gynecologist." Instead of a standard hysteroscopy, which uses carbon dioxide to distend the cervix and a hysteroscope that is five millimeters wide, the mini-hysteroscopy uses a watery substance for distension and a hysteroscope that is only 3.3 millimeters wide. The smaller device is less painful than the standard one, especially for insertion and removal, and the mini-hysteroscopy overall requires less hardware.[7]

Ombelet and his colleagues also advocate for education in fertility medicine to increase the number of IVF clinics in underserviced areas of the world. The lack of education and training in laboratory practices and reproductive medicine hinders clinic expansion in many parts of the world. The fact that IVF education and service provision are most advanced in former colonial states and least advanced in former colonized states is not lost on anyone in the fertility industry, especially in under-resourced countries. The medical anthropologist Trudie Gerrits notes that "training in this specialized field of assisted reproductive technologies—both the clinical and embryological part—is not offered in Ghana, which means that embryologists' expertise and skills in particular are a scarce and precious commodity. . . . The Ghanaian local assisted reproductive technology industry cannot function without this new 'neocolonial dependency.'"[8] Skilled technicians are just as essential as proper tools and infrastructure to make IVF clinics in underserved areas possible.

Historical Technologies Will Stay Relevant

Child-seekers will continue to use less advanced technologies alongside technologies that require advanced medical assistance and infrastructures. Technologies and methods with historical longevity, such as fertility calendars and home-based insemination, will coexist alongside advances in high-technology methods. Home-based insemination persists especially in countries where access to ARTs is restricted or illegal for some identity groups (usually gay, trans, non-binary, and lesbian individuals). They may find assistance in printed or Internet guides to doing so, which originate in the feminist women's health movements of the 1970s. Lesbian insemination guidebooks have been in

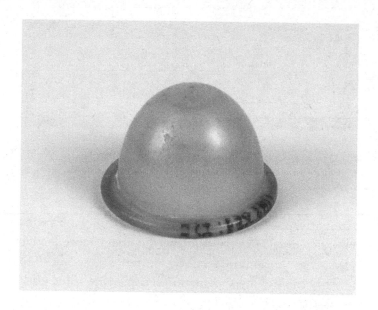

Figure 9 Though IVF and its successor technologies dominated discussions of fertility technology in popular culture from the late 1970s forward, those legally excluded from accessing high-tech methods instead used lower-tech methods with historical longevity, like cervical caps and syringes. Cervical cap, c. 1982. *Source:* Courtesy National Museum of American History, Smithsonian Institution, Washington, DC.

print since 1979, and syringes, cannulas, cervical caps or diaphragms, eye droppers, and jars are available to anyone who purchases them from a medical supply store or online.[9]

Furthermore, some women's and lesbian health organizations have maintained their own sperm banks and

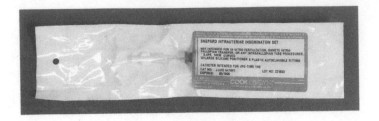

Figure 10 Shepard Intrauterine Insemination Set, c. 1996. *Source:* Courtesy National Museum of American History, Smithsonian Institution, Washington, DC.

alternative-insemination services. Such organizations may also provide initial information about reproductive physiology, including fertility awareness methods, to identify the timing of ovulation. People who want fertility assistance, but on their own terms, choose methods that do not violate their own boundaries. They develop "hybrid-technology practices," as Laura Mamo calls them, or practices of borrowing from both high- and low-tech methods according to their own health and preferences. To take one example, one couple that she interviewed did not want to use hormonal drugs at first but accepted them later: "We progressed through cervical-cap inseminations with no ovarian stimulation to Clomid with intrauterine stimulation to Pergonal or FSH [follicle-stimulating hormone] injectibles with either cervical cap or intrauterine insemination and eventually to IVF."[10] Individuals and couples have a range of options for charting their own journeys through the fertility landscape—as long as they have the time, patience, finances, and good health to do so.

Ovulation timing is another low-tech method that continues to have relevance and legitimacy for heterosexual couples. Two Melbourne, Australia-based physicians, the husband-and-wife team John Billings (1918–2007) and Evelyn Livingston Billings (1918–2013), were popular promoters of a Roman Catholic Church–approved method from 1953 through the 2000s. In the 1960s and 1970s, they toured the world teaching the Billings ovulation method. It involved checking secretions of the cervical mucus daily for the changes in thickness that indicated ovulation was forthcoming. The Church's current natural family planning (NFP) program supports couples using basal body temperature (BBT), cervical mucus measurement, over-the-counter ovulation predictor kits that measure hormonal changes, or all three as fertility management tools.[11]

In the 1970s, as members of the second-wave feminist movement and international women's health movement explored alternatives to standardized drug-based medical care, they sought drug- and doctor's-office-free methods of managing fertility. As their motivation to learn the method stemmed from a desire to live a drug-free lifestyle, not to adhere to religious teachings, Billings method and NFP instructors were sometimes reluctant to share their knowledge with non-Catholic women. The nonreligious fertility awareness activist Katie Singer outlined her own difficulties trying to learn the method in 1997, wondering, "Are the teaching methods, commitments, and self-control expressed in the Catholic community not available to others?"[12] Despite encountering resistance from the Catholic laypersons leading the sessions, Singer successfully learned non-hormonal methods in order to feel closer to the natural rhythms of the earth and sky and to connect more intimately with her partner.

NFP is an example of a method with supplementary technologies, like ovulation predictor kits and thermometers, that people can use to promote (or to restrict) fertility from markedly diverse spiritual frameworks. In 1995, the public health practitioner Toni Weschler published a how-to guide to a secular version of NFP that she called the fertility awareness method (FAM). FAM involved a mixture of calendar, mucus, and BBT methods. There were two differences between NFP and FAM, though: first, FAM users can use condoms or other barrier methods during fertile periods if attempting to avoid pregnancy. Second, Weschler recommends examining the cervix with the fingers, as it noticeably changes shape and texture around ovulation. One of Weschler's motivations for writing the guidebook was skepticism toward for-profit medicine, and she argued that managing fertility through FAM was one way to lessen visits to the gynecologist's office or to avoid them altogether.[13]

Another way that tracking methods have been updated in the twenty-first century is through the development of smartphone apps. As of 2019, there were 200 fertility tracking apps available for Android or iOS smartphones. Menstrual tracking and fertility management apps are part of a larger shift in the use of smartphones to track personal health and wellness goals. These apps most often correlate user's input with Ogino-Knaus calendar methods to determine when the user is fertile or not. Some allow the user to input fertility-awareness information on cervical fluid and urinary lutenizing hormones, but the apps do not include that information in their algorithms.[14]

Some apps come with their own thermometer that can be plugged directly into a smartphone. Companies make their algorithm available to users through a variety of products and connect each of them with a smartphone app. For example, Valley Electronics' Daysy algorithm is based on a combination of Ogino-Knaus calendar timing, the user's BBT, and the inputted data of previous users. The accuracy of the data for each user depends to some extent on how much related data (such as body mass index, or BMI) the user inputs, and it is not clear where or for how long the personal data is stored.[15]

Wearable body-monitoring technology called "smart jewelry" serves a similar function as tracking apps, though it tracks the wearer's menstrual cycle, heart rate, breathing, and sleep automatically. Though apps and smart jewelry are marketed as empowering wearers to understand their bodies better, and to help wearers plan or avoid pregnancy, "these technologies do not necessarily mean reproductive decisions are any easier to make, especially if a woman does not have a partner or the economic resources required to engage in further fertility interventions such as egg freezing." Although sometimes partners were involved in the tracking processes, "this was usually intermittent and often involved women appealing to their interest in technology, data, and/or the timing of sex." Despite empowering rhetoric, fertility tracking apps and wearable jewelry place the emotional labor of planning or avoiding conception squarely on the partner capable of pregnancy, reproducing "entrenched gendered responsibilities for conception and emotional labor."[16]

Low-Tech IVF

Even after more than forty years of IVF and with advancements such as ICSI, the success rate as measured in live births per embryo transfer is still variable, according to age and health factors. For example, the success rate of IVF per embryo transfer in the United States in 2018 was 12 percent for patients over forty-three years old and 48 percent for those under thirty-five.[17] Individuals and couples may try processes that make IVF simpler and reduce its cost, such as the INVOcell device and the Walking Egg Project, both used for intravaginal culture (IVC).

INVOcell is a thimble-sized acrylic device that enables fertilization and early embryo development to take place in the vaginal cavity, rather than in a laboratory dish. The French embryologist Claude Ranoux published the results of initial experiments with his handmade version of the device in 1988, and the US Food and Drug Administration approved it in 2015 for commercial manufacturing. The patient first takes standard ovarian stimulation hormones. The physician removes the eggs and then combines the eggs and donor or partner sperm in the device. After the device incubates in the vagina for five days, the physician removes it and checks if any of the eggs were fertilized. If so, one or more blastocysts are then implanted in the uterus. A March 2021 study with 463 patients undergoing 526 cycles at five US clinics had a 19–34 percent rate of viable blastocysts per cycle. The live birth rate after the blastocysts were transferred was between 40 and 61 percent, depending on the patient's age, weight, ovarian reserve, and their partner's level of male factor infertility. In that study, the live birth rate was comparable to that of traditional IVF, though the number of blastocysts formed for subsequent implantation was not as high.[18]

The Walking Egg lab method is another simplified method of IVF culturing. It does not require anesthesia, incubation equipment, or the expensive infrastructure of

IVF laboratories. For insemination of the egg, the sperm is washed and only 1,000–10,000 sperm are placed in a tube with the oocyte. Then, the Walking Egg lab method can either involve incubation in an equilibrated acid-base-water solution alongside a culture medium or incubation with the tube interiorly: "A tube filled with culture medium containing the oocytes and washed spermatozoa is hermetically closed and placed in the vagina. It is held intravaginally by a diaphragm for incubation for 44–50 hours." The tube is then removed and inspected to see if the egg is fertilized. If so, the physician can then transfer the embryo to the uterus for implantation, and the procedure "can avoid many problems frequently occurring in regular IVF laboratories, such as unwanted temperature changes [and] air quality problems." The first baby conceived with the Walking Egg lab method was born in Ghana in August 2017.[19]

Fertilization inside the body has advantages and disadvantages compared to traditional IVF. The advantages are that it is much less expensive per IVF cycle (US$6,800 as compared to US$15,000–20,000 in 2017), it takes fewer physician visits, and not as many eggs are retrieved, so the patient takes fewer stimulating hormones. This is a shift in perspective from fertility medicine in the 1980s, which had a more-is-better perspective regarding egg retrieval. Furthermore, fertility medicine specialists can learn the method quickly and use it in parts of the world that do not have the technical infrastructure for more high-tech processes. The main disadvantages are that clinicians and laboratory workers can neither monitor the fertilization process nor pinpoint problems until after the device is removed, and that it works less well for women with a body mass index (BMI) over 35 or who are over thirty-eight years old. Another study suggested that INVOcell could be combined with ICSI, highlighting the likelihood that combinations of IVF-related technologies and processes to improve rates of implantation will continue in the future.[20]

Low-tech processes like INVOcell and the Walking Egg lab method will continue to exist alongside high-tech processes such as time-lapse imaging, closing access gaps between high-income and low-income child-seekers. Like other fertility technologies, low-tech processes address some problems (cost, time commitment, and hormone stimulation) but not others (age, weight, or health problems such as polycystic ovary syndrome). For some seekers, though, there is no price too high to pay for a child of their own.

Add-Ons: Time-Lapse Imaging

Like many areas of medicine, reproductive medicine attracts inventors and entrepreneurs. Some of their solutions may provide valid diagnostic information or improve

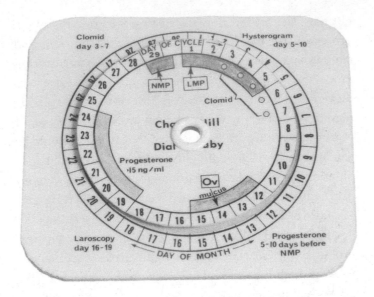

Figure 11 High-tech methods like IVF include historical references like this IVF Calculation Disc, 2005. *Source:* Courtesy Museum of Contraception and Reproduction, Vienna.

chances of pregnancy but are not yet tested or approved by medical regulatory bodies. Some can be added to standard IVF treatments or are offered as part of comprehensive fertility medicine packages that may not be necessary for all patients. These add-ons can be problematic, as "IVF patients may not be adequately informed about the benefits and risk of IVF add-ons or may not be aware of the paucity of supportive evidence for safety and effectiveness."[21] As navigating the world of add-ons may be confusing even for knowledgeable clients, some countries' regulatory bodies provide guidance. The UK's Human Fertilisation and Embryology Authority (HFEA) publishes a traffic-light system, which rates add-ons according to available cost implications, risks, and evidence. A green light indicates that a treatment has shown positive results according to at least one randomized control study, an amber light indicates mixed results, and a red light indicates no positive results.[22] Reviews of add-ons available since 2015 show their overall limited benefit and potential unknown harms to patients.

A survey taken in June and July 2020 showed that up to twenty-four add-ons were available at clinics across Australia, many of which mirrored those available in the UK. They ranged from mild and complementary (aspirin, acupuncture) to loosely linked (melatonin) to highly technological (assisted hatching). Another review of ten add-ons, from screening hysteroscopy (examination of the uterus under anesthesia) to androgen supplements, found either that they had no effect on implantation or live birth rates or that there was insufficient data to support such a claim. A third review of five add-ons solely for the endometrium (mucus membrane lining the uterus) showed that their effects ranged from unclear (vasodilators such as sildenafil [Viagra] to thicken the endometrium) to harmful (endometrial scratching, which inflames the endometrium and might make the embryo more likely to implant).

These reviews caution that profit may motivate clinics "to provide costly IVF add-ons with no evidence base."[23]

One of the add-ons that has received the most attention from scholars and fertility medicine specialists is time-lapse imaging, and as such, it is valuable to examine its implications in detail. Time-lapse imaging of embryos from fertilization to three days afterward (for double embryo transfer) to five days afterward (for single embryo transfer) is designed to help embryologists choose the healthiest possible embryo for implantation. Time-lapse imaging technologies "allow for continuous observation by taking photographs every 5 to 20 minutes while the embryos remain in the incubator. . . . By matching the videos with growth patterns of embryos that developed into healthy fetuses, the time-lapse system suggests which embryos are most likely to grow into a baby." The time-lapse systems film the developing embryos and quantify the visual information onto grids, and then clinicians must have specialized training in algorithmic analysis to predict each one's likelihood of turning into a blastocyst. These systems, called EmbryoScope (manufactured by Vitrolife) and Eeva (short for Early Embryo Viability Assessment, manufactured by Merck), depend on past selections to predict future embryo viability. In a May 2019 survey of fertility clinic websites in the United Kingdom, time-lapse imaging costs an average of £478 as a stand-alone treatment and an average of £4,020 as part of a treatment package. The systems themselves cost clinics £75,000–80,000.[24]

Time-lapse imaging alters more than just the process of embryo selection. As Lucy van de Wiel writes, "by matching the embryos' cellular growth patterns to previous embryonic populations' recorded developmental rhythms, time-lapse technology brings embryonic aging to the forefront in embryo selection." Time-lapse imaging turns embryo selection into a "new, data-driven way of seeing" using "automated pattern recognition and algorithmic predictive analysis."[25] This process not only changes how laboratory technicians and embryologists see and choose embryos for implantation, but it also changes how a prospective parent or parents see their embryos: "ranking means that the woman or couple has a *quantified* sense of the blastocyst's potential for development."[26]

The datafication of embryo selection has consequences not only for current patients but also for future patients, clinic staff, and the companies that harvest, store, and manipulate the inputted embryonic data. Clinic staff use patient data aggregated from the past in order to make decisions about the viability of the embryos in the present, but not all staff members always grade the similar embryos the same way, introducing further uncertainty into the process. If past decisions about selected embryos were in error, then those errors appear incorrectly as positive traits. Sometime in the future, even the embryo selection process could be automated, using machine learning and artificial intelligence; indeed, "the introduction of artificial intelligence in artificial reproduction is thus currently giving rise to new clinical and research practices." Embedding embryo selection in data systems that connect pharmaceutical, biotech, and fertility companies deepens the data relationships within the fertility industry; supports the development of algorithms as salable products themselves, complementing "the new reproductive data infrastructures established through the growing sales of time-lapse systems"; and further embeds child-seekers (and their abstracted data) in the world of high-tech fertility management.[27]

HFEA gives time-lapse imaging an amber light, as "being undisturbed while they grow may improve the quality of the embryos but there's certainly not enough evidence to show that time-lapse incubation and imaging is effective at improving your chance of having a baby." Before getting a green light from HFEA and other national regulatory agencies, time-lapse imaging needs more proof to support Vitrolife's and Merck's claims that their products improve embryo selection.[28] In general, inventors and suppliers of new add-ons may be pursuing not only patient satisfaction and profit but also the satisfaction of developing an IVF breakthrough technology to improve implantation and live-birth success rates markedly.[29]

In Vitro Maturation and MDNA Transplantation

Some of the other high-technology methods currently being researched include in vitro maturation (IVM), which retrieves "immature oocytes directly from the ovaries through a procedure using fine-needle aspiration. They would then be matured in vitro before being fertilized through standard IVF." Another is obtaining functional gametes from other types of cells—either human embryonic stem cells (ESC) or induced pluripotent stem cells (iPSC); and the use of mitochondrial DNA from a donor egg to manifest so-called three-parent embryos. For the latter, "women with healthy mitochondrial histories are asked to donate their eggs to women with family histories of disease, and the recipients' nuclear genetic material is transferred to the healthy egg. This enables the recipient to conceive a child who is genetically her own, if the terms of genetics are limited to nuclear DNA."[30] The embryo is then the product of three people's gametes, containing the nuclear DNA of the intending parents and the mitochondrial DNA of an egg donor. The UK's Human Fertilisation and Embryology Act (1990) was amended in 2015 to legalize this procedure, called MDNA transplantation; the United Kingdom is the only country that permits it.

The procedure is intended to help women with mitochondrial disorders (often undetectable in PGD testing) avoid passing those disorders onto potential children, and to ensure that those children are their genetic offspring. Unfortunately for the further acceptance of this procedure, "most maternally inherited mitochondrial disorders only develop in adulthood, whereas mitochondrial disorders that severely affect babies are caused, in approximately 80% of cases, by nuclear defects that are inherited from both parents." In other words, replacing mitochondrial DNA alone cannot prevent diseases inherited from both parents, and the procedure helps only in the 20 percent of diseases that are only inherited maternally. The procedure also carries further risks:

> [1] the potential side-effects caused by the co-existence of two different types of mitochondria within the embryo's cytoplasm, including the possible carry-over of pathogenic mtDNA; [2] the possible defects caused by mismatching the nuclear and mitochondrial genomes, such as metabolic dysfunction and epigenetics effects; and [3] the social and psychological consequences of having been conceived using genetic material from three people.[31]

Access to the procedure is heavily restricted, and disorders can often be found in gametes more easily and cost-efficiently using an older diagnosis method, PGT. The ethical considerations of procedures like IVM and MDNA leave many open questions about their use, especially if more problems with them are identified and more countries legalize them.

Uterine Transplants

Another significant technological step is IVF in persons with transplanted uteri. The first modern attempt at a uterine transplant alone took place in Saudi Arabia in 2000. The first IVF procedure in a transplanted uterus from a live donor that resulted in a live birth happened fourteen years later in Gothenburg, Sweden. The first live birth via IVF in a uterine transplant in the United States occurred in 2017, and the IVF-transplant procedure has resulted in seventy uterine transfers with fourteen live births worldwide as of June 2021. Uterine transplants have been a focus of reproductive medical attention in the last two decades because "uterus transplantation is the only known treatment for women suffering from uterus factor infertility, and thus the immediate purpose of the procedure would be to restore fertility to patients with an abnormal, damaged, or absent uterus."[32] If the transplant is successful, the donated uterus is removed after a certain period of time and number of successful IVF pregnancies a number that the patient would determine.

Uterine transplantation is an intricate procedure, involving immunosuppressant drug regimens, the risk of organ rejection, the possible development of a thrombosis, and other complications. Connecting the blood vessels of the donated uterus to those in the recipient's body is particularly tricky. But there are many other steps before the transplant and IVF can begin. On the practical side, there is no uterine donation registry, so in the case of live donation, the person without a uterus must ask a prospective donor for theirs (or the prospective donor must offer). Transplantation from a nondirected (anonymous) living donor or a deceased donor is also possible, though familial donors with identical blood types lower the risk of rejection. For some studies, prospective transplant recipients must secure their own donor. Interviews with ten uterus-seekers in Sweden described how they reached out to their mothers as well as older sisters or aunts, raising the possibility that they could gestate a child using the same uterus in which they themselves were gestated. The emotional intricacy of asking (and possibly receiving) an organ donation in this situation is obvious.[33]

Familial complexities aside, IVF in uterine transplants sparks the possibility of gestating pregnancies outside the human body completely in artificial wombs (ectogenesis). Research on human ectogenesis is still illegal in the United Kingdom, but animal research has been in progress there since the early 1960s. For humans, "technology that can mimic the functions of the maternal uterus can help save the lives of extremely premature babies born on the cusp of viability. . . . Such technology can also help women who suffer from uterus factor infertility and thus are unable to gestate their own child." Research is underway in Sweden (by the same team that facilitated the first uterine transplant) to create a viable bioengineered uterus, including artificial amniotic fluid and an artificial endometrium. A bioengineered uterus could also be used for part of a pregnancy; for example, gestation could begin in the human womb, with the fetus transferred later to the artificial one. Successful human ectogenesis, whether wholly or partially gestated in an artificial uterus, could open up a new world of possibilities of reproduction.[34]

Farther in the future is in vitro gametogenesis (IVG), the creation of gametes using pluripotent stem cells (cells that can differentiate into many cell types). If a patient cannot provide gametes for an assisted reproduction treatment, IVG could create gametes from their skin cells. "Artificial gametes . . . raise 'one of the most dramatic possibilities that two men (and maybe also two women) could create a baby that is genetically related [to] both of them, in the same way as men and women.' Artificial gametes widen procreative possibilities for those unable to reproduce via traditional methods of sexual reproduction." As a result, a couple of any gender could provide all the gametes needed to produce an embryo that is genetically related to both of them.[35]

Transgender and Non-Binary Pregnancy

Transgender and non-binary individuals use gamete storage, AI, and IVF treatments in some different ways than cisgender individuals. The hormone therapy and surgeries that transgender individuals in some countries still must move through to receive legal recognition of their gender status renders them sterile. This requirement is starting to change—for example, as of 2013, Swedish law no longer requires sterility for granting legal gender recognition. However, in many countries, transgender people need to preserve their gametes before hormonal treatments and gender confirmation surgery if they want to have genetically related children in the future. Young transgender persons may want to freeze gametes before beginning hormone treatment, but in countries like the United Kingdom, doing so may be cost-prohibitive or simply unavailable. So, "it is therefore not surprising that young people prioritize their pubertal changes over gamete storage, particularly when parenting is not top of the list for most adolescents."[36]

In a similar vein, non-binary individuals assigned female at birth (AFAB) and individuals assigned male at birth (AMAB) have to time conception, pregnancy, and gender confirmation carefully. Interviews with five AFAB non-binary individuals in Canada who wanted to gestate and to give birth showed how they "consciously considered how to balance their medical and social transitions with their reproductive goals." Simultaneous gender confirmation and pregnancy was challenging from medical, legal, and social points of view, and so they had to choose whether to undergo gender confirmation or become pregnant first. As one interviewee put it, "It feels like you can't do the two at the same time . . . you're kind of compromising one way or the other . . . like obviously I can't physically transition at the same time as I'm pregnant because that's medically contraindicated." AMAB individuals who take androgen blockers may have reduced sperm quality, as anti-androgens "inhibit the action of testosterone, removing the downstream effects of testosterone including spermatogenesis and maintenance of the mature testicle." They may have to stop anti-androgens to have healthy sperm for conception.[37]

Non-binary, trans, and queer individuals in the United States have institutional support from the Ethics Committee of the American Society for Reproductive Medicine (ASRM)—the principal professional organization for fertility medicine—to forward their interests in having children. The Ethics Committee recommended in 2013 that lesbians, gay men, and single people of any orientation have the right to be parents and to seek fertility treatment. In 2015, they recommended that transgender people be allowed treatment, as "transgender persons have the same interests as other persons in having children and in accessing fertility services for fertility preservation and reproduction." A survey with fifty-one men, trans/masculine, or non-binary people in English-speaking countries confirmed ASRM's statement and found that "the routinization of conception serves to further normalize the lives of gestational parents who are men, trans/masculine, or non-binary, as well as their families," and that "fertility clinics have an important role to play in normalizing and affirming [their] conception-related needs." Most of them became pregnant via known donors or with their partner's gametes, and for them, "conception was a positive and straightforward experience."[38] Normalcy, in these cases, was a comfort.

In the future, uterine transplants paired with IVF make pregnancy a possibility for transgender women or cisgender men as well. The availability of uterine transplants, along with pregnancies in transgender and non-binary individuals, alters traditional categories of parenthood in a male-female gender binary. In short, "reproductive technologies are increasingly allowing us to separate genetic, gestational, and social parenthood."[39]

For-Profit Fertility

Private fertility technology companies are being established more and more often as a means for investor profit and less for altruistic reasons. Leaders of such companies also want to make the processes of egg freezing, IVF, and implantation more accessible and less expensive by automating them. Fertility entrepreneurs like Martín Varsavsky want to automate the processes of egg freezing and IVF using a now-prototype machine called NaturaLife, which replaces embryologists with "robotics, biochips, and A.I. technology." NaturaLife "would perform the same functions as a human embryologist—select sperm and eggs to create embryos and then genetically test them—with greater accuracy and at a fraction of the cost."[40] That cost, of course, being the salary and benefits for a professional embryologist.

The array of fertility management possibilities can be bewildering, so some companies offer their services in packages. To take one example, Prelude Fertility's "Prelude Method" "proposes a streamlined approach to fertility management that combines egg freezing with a predefined treatment trajectory that spans an extended time during the reproductive life course and beyond." The Prelude Method is a package that includes egg freezing, sperm freezing, genetic testing (probably PGT-A), embryo fertilization, and single embryo transfer. To take another, Progyny streamlines egg freezing into a long-term treatment package with its SMART (Science and Member-Driven Assisted Reproductive Technology) Cycle. This package covers consultations, tests, and infertility treatments, such as egg freezing, intra-cytoplasmic sperm injection (ICSI), assisted hatching, and genetic selection technologies (PGT-A) for single embryo transfer.[41] However, some of these add-ons, like assisted hatching, have unproven value and may simply be unnecessary for the success of an IVF cycle.

These packages reduce clients' uncertainty regarding what services they need, placing them on "a technologically mediated reproductive life course" governed by the availability of technology (and the ability to pay for it). They target younger clients and embed them in a specific articulation of biomedical fertility management over a lifetime: contraception and egg freezing in one's twenties followed by egg thawing, IVF, and multiple add-ons in one's thirties or early forties. In other words, individuals "may now physically and financially invest in simultaneously preventing conception with contraceptive pharmaceuticals and ensuring continued fertility with egg freezing. . . . As egg freezing practices expand the target group for assisted reproduction, so embryo selection technologies expand the IVF cycle with additional steps and investments."[42]

The COVID-19 pandemic exacerbated many people's concerns about their own health and the health of their potential future offspring, leading to an increase in demand for egg freezing services from summer 2020 through the first half of 2021, at least. One US-based for-profit fertility company, Kindbody, supplements one of its brick-and-mortar clinics with a mobile clinic and organizes pop-up events available at some companies that cover its services via employee insurance plans.[43] The long-term effect of the pandemic on the global for-profit fertility industry cannot yet be determined. Those who lead and manage fertility companies see fertility as a good investment—especially in countries with few regulations, like the United States—and as a growth industry. In conclusion, potential clients should look closely at the fine print of any package before signing on the dotted line.

This journey through fertility technology from the 1850s through the present illustrates how the four themes in the introduction have intersected over time. First, the political and legal status of fertility technology in different countries shows that inequalities in national economies, infrastructures, and gendered power perpetuate inequalities in access to, and use of, fertility technology. Though some of the clearest forms of abuse have been curtailed, as in the example of the Australian couple hiring a Thai surrogate and abandoning a boy with Down syndrome, the fact remains that citizens of under-resourced and developing countries often serve as surrogates or egg donors for citizens of wealthier countries. Those living in developing countries who have the financial means to use fertility services but no access to them must travel to countries where these services are available. The wealthiest potential users, often employed at major corporations, are encouraged to develop fertility management plans that include IVF and

The growth of fertility as a for-profit industry may lead to people making decisions that are not in their own best interests.

an ever-increasing number of costly and often unproven add-ons beginning in their twenties. However, the growth of fertility as a for-profit industry, especially in under-regulated countries, along with the idea that the timing of childbearing should align with an employer's labor requirements, may lead to people making decisions that are not in their own best interests. They may also buy more services and undergo more treatments than they actually need.

Second, fertility technology illuminates key moments in the histories of women, gender, and sexuality. On the one side, the use of fertility technology in a heterosexual marriage can uphold binary gender norms and strengthen connections between motherhood and womanhood, specifically via the idea that gestating and giving birth to a child makes one a genuine woman and a mother (even if there is no genetic connection). The historical and contemporary precepts of Roman Catholicism, Judaism, and Sunni and Shia Islam all reinforce these connections to one degree or another. On the other, the use of fertility technology may make conception, gestation, and birth possible for individuals who intentionally use it to queer dualistic notions of gender and reproduction. IVF for non-binary, transgender, and genderqueer people, not to mention IVF with transplanted uteri, makes pregnancy across and beyond genders a possibility. Scholars, medical practitioners, and clinic staff must "begin to disentangle gender from the acts of conception, pregnancy, and birth."[44]

Third, technologies for fertility diagnosis and treatment show that both kinds of technology are necessary for making conception possible. There is no need to treat a condition that does not in fact impede fertility or is misidentified. Diagnostic techniques have expanded focus over the period covered in this book, from the bodies in which pregnancy occurs to analysis of sperm under a microscope to the embryos tested by PGT-A for genetic abnormalities and observed in time-lapse imaging systems. Salpingograms and insufflation machines could, and still do, identify blockages in the fallopian tubes that impede the travel of sperm to egg. Treatments that address and heighten the possibility of conception do just that, though their effectiveness may be hampered if the original diagnosis is incorrect. They do not necessarily cure or solve fertility problems per se. The latest treatments designed to improve on IVF with ICSI—most recently, add-ons like time-lapse imaging—are often hurried to a consumer market anxious for children and willing to overlook (or at least to accept) their unverified value. Manifesting a pregnancy from conception to live birth is a process that can still resist the most sophisticated diagnostic and treatment efforts available.

Fourth, fertility and contraceptive technologies are often the same procedures and devices. They are studied separately from menstrual technologies as well, though of course they all relate to one another depending on one's desire (or not) for pregnancy and place in the reproductive lifecycle. While books like this one treat these technologies in separate categories—indeed, there is a previous book in this series on contraception—rarely are they as separable as scholars make them out to be. In particular, the simplest and least expensive devices (cervical caps and condoms) and techniques (tracking ovulation timing) can be used for both conception and contraception, pointing to their versatility and the need for scholars to study them together as part of a wide spectrum of reproductive technologies.[45]

In summary, a history of fertility technologies can only hint at the vastly complex ways that the desire for children affects the lives of individuals, couples, communities, and nations. The technologies that make pregnancy possible for some people are a source of disappointment for others. They are means of giving certain embryos a chance to develop as persons in the world, but also a means of keeping other embryos and potential persons out of the world. Fertility technologies are much more than a way to address reproductive health problems or "simply a medical procedure to cure a medically described condition." They are "a tool through which people create people."[46] How they will develop next   and what kinds of human life will emerge as a result of using them—remains to be seen.

POSTSCRIPT

New Realities after *Dobbs*

I finished revisions on this book in late April 2022. Its page proofs were printed for my review on June 24, 2022, coincidentally the same day that the US Supreme Court handed down a 6–3 decision in *Dobbs v. Jackson Women's Health Organization,* which held that the Constitution does not confer the right to an abortion. The decision is an intentional regression of the right to bodily autonomy and to access health care, not to mention a deliberate blow against the principles of reproductive justice. Rights to privacy, contraception, and the free choice of marriage partner may be threatened in the future as well.

Dobbs will have a momentous and long-lasting effect on the use of reproductive technologies in the United States. For example, legislators in some states have now introduced bills that give embryos the legal rights of human beings. If those bills become law, discarding unused embryos created during IVF may be categorized as abortions: criminal acts.

As this book has shown, though, when a country reduces or forbids access to fertility technologies and procedures—or its citizens have limited access to them due to the absence of infrastructure—those circumstances do not change its citizens' desires for children. Rather, those in the United States who wish to become biological parents might redirect their approaches to fertility and increasingly turn toward low-tech fertility methods that do not produce extra embryos, such as AI with donor sperm. Those who can afford it (and have the legal right to do so) may undergo IVF, gestate, and give birth in countries where abortion is legal in case of complications. Or, they may seek surrogates outside the United States who have the right to abort ectopic pregnancies or pregnancies that otherwise risk the surrogates' health or life.

The *Dobbs* decision, in short, reaches beyond US borders. It has global ramifications not only for Americans, but also for the international reproductive technology industry. It is up to everyone who supports reproductive justice to ensure that this new global reproscape upholds the health, safety, and dignity of all involved as would-be parents seek to build families in this uncertain world.

ACKNOWLEDGMENTS

I am grateful to Katie Helke and Laura Keeler at the MIT Press and the expertise of the four reviewers: Christina Weis, Kelly O'Donnell, Gayle Davis, and Kylie Baldwin, for their professional support. Doris Lampert and the interlibrary loan staff at Technische Universität Darmstadt facilitated the delivery of numerous critical books to my desk from across Germany, and Christoph Merkelbach's leadership made pandemic-era work the best experience that it could be. Jessica Murphy (Center for the History of Medicine, Francis A. Countway Library of Medicine, Harvard University) and Kay Peterson (National Museum of American History, Smithsonian Institution) assisted me with illustrations, and it is a pleasure to reprint Paula Knight's work with her permission. Stine Willum Adrian, Olivia Fischer, Alina Geampana, Sarah Lensen, and Damien Riggs kindly shared their published and unpublished work with me. Many friends and family members contributed behind-the-scenes support as well: Dagmar Bellmann, Tobias Boll, Michele Campbell, Kate Costello, Michelle Cunningham-Wandel, Stefan Glatzl, Mar Hicks, Corinna Norrick-Rühl, Lora Stephan, and Shalini Wittstruck; not to mention Adrienne Drucker, Alan Drucker, Diane K. Drucker, Donald S. Drucker, Joey Drucker, Jory Drucker Mangurten, Betty Watson, the late Chuck Watson, and Katie Watson. This book is dedicated to the memory of Chuck Watson, who always believed in me.

ACKNOWLEDGMENTS

GLOSSARY

Artificial insemination (AI) (by donor [**AID**], by husband [**AIH**], also **intravaginal insemination** [**IVI**], **intracervical insemination** [**ICI**], and **intrauterine insemination** [**IUI**])

The use of a syringe and cannula to place seminal fluid into the vagina, cervix, or uterus. Seminal fluid is ejaculated, transferred into a jar or other small container, then siphoned into the syringe with a cannula placed at one end. The cannula is placed as deep inside the vaginal canal toward the cervix as possible. The seminal fluid can come from a patient's partner, a known donor, or an anonymous donor, and sometimes in the past when the partner had a low sperm count, donor and husband sperm was mixed together to blur the identity of the child.

Assisted reproductive technologies (ARTs), also **new reproductive technologies (NRTs)**

The umbrella term for the technologies and medical processes surrounding removing an egg from a woman's body, fertilizing it with sperm in a laboratory, and either returning the fertilized egg to the same woman's body or placing it in the body of a donor. Technologies used to supplement IVF are called adjuncts or add-ons.

Azoospermia

The absence of spermatozoa from seminal fluid—in the context of fertility technology, a diagnosis of azoospermia indicates the need for an alternate source of sperm in order to make a pregnancy possible.

Cryopreservation

The preservation of tissue at extremely low temperatures—in the context of fertility technology, the preservation of human eggs, sperm, or embryos.

Egg, sperm, and embryo banks (also cryobanks)

Facilities for the preservation of human reproductive tissues at extremely low temperatures. Sperm banks were first established in Iowa in the 1950s. Embryo and egg banks proliferated in the 2000s after the development of the Cryotop (a thin strip of film for preserving frozen tissues) for vitrification of human tissue in Japan.

Fertility traveler

A person who travels to a different country to participate in fertility treatment, either for themselves or as a provider, usually an egg provider (also known as traveling egg providers).

Gamete intrafallopian transfer (GIFT)

A procedure developed by Ricardo Asch in San Antonio, Texas, in 1984, in which eggs and sperm are removed from the donors' bodies but replaced into the fallopian tubes so that they fertilize on their own. It is less likely to succeed than IVF and is used only in cases where couples have a religious or moral objection to fertilization outside the body.

Hysterosalpingography

A procedure for the determination of blockages in the fallopian tubes or abnormalities in the uterus. After the patient lies down under a fluoroscope (X-ray imager), liquid containing iodine is injected into the uterus, and any blockages or abnormalities are visible by contrast through the fluoroscope's image capture.

Intracytoplasmic sperm injection (ICSI)

A specialized form of IVF developed in Belgium in 1992, in which a single sperm is inserted into an oocyte. It is especially useful in cases where the amount and/or quality of sperm is low. After the oocyte is fertilized, it is left to mature in an incubator before being placed in the uterus.

In vitro fertilization (IVF)

A series of medical procedures leading to the implantation of an externally fertilized oocyte into the uterus, from which the first live human birth occurred in 1978. First, a woman takes a hormone-suppressing drug for roughly three weeks, followed by an ovarian stimulation drug such as Pergonal. Next, the partner's (or donor's) sperm is washed (cleaned of any chemicals or impurities), and eggs are aspirated from the woman's uterus. Then, eggs are fertilized (possibly only with a single sperm, as in ICSI), and the fertilized embryos may be examined through PGD or PGT-A. A few weeks after one or more of the embryos is transferred to the uterus, the woman will take a pregnancy test to see if the embryos have implanted.

Laparoscopy

A minimally invasive pelvic or abdominal operation using a laparoscope, a thin probe with a camera and/or light on its end. Such surgery requires only a small incision and local anesthetic. In the fertility technology context, it is used as a diagnostic tool to determine fallopian tube blockages and for tubal ligation; English physician Patrick Steptoe made its use popular for egg retrieval in IVF procedures.

Laparotomy

A surgical operation in which the abdomen is opened, and the internal organs are checked for disease or injury. In the fertility technology context, it was used as a tool to diagnose fertility problems and for tubal ligation before the development of the less-invasive laparoscopy technique.

Ogino-Knaus ovulation timing

Kyusaku Ogino (Japan) and Hermann H. Knaus (Austria) independently confirmed the timing of ovulation in 1923 and in 1929, respectively. Their findings, jointly called Ogino-Knaus, provided the foundation for calendar-based timing methods that couples could use to encourage or to avoid a pregnancy. Different versions of these timing methods are known as the rhythm method, the Billings method, natural family planning (NFP), and the fertility awareness method (FAM).

Preimplantation genetic diagnosis (PGD), preimplantation genetic screening (PGS), and preimplantation genetic testing for aneuploidy (PGT-A)

PGD is the process of conducting biopsies and tests on embryos to determine sex and the presence of any molecular, hereditary disease before implantation. PGS is a now-unused term for PGT-A, in which embryos are biopsied and pre-screened for chromosomal abnormalities before implantation, potentially to decrease rates of miscarriages and to increase chances of live births.

Selective reproductive technologies (SRTs)

An umbrella term defined in 2014 by Tine M. Gammeltoft and Ayo Wahlberg as technologies that are "not only used to prevent certain kinds of children from being born . . . [but that] can also help bring specific kinds of children into the world through the selective fertilization of gametes or implantation of embryos." They include elements of now-standard ART procedures, such as PGD and PGT-A, or more controversial procedures, such as embryo sex selection or the creation of "savior siblings" for existing children needing cord blood or bone marrow donors.

Technosemen

A term put forward by Matthew Schmidt and Lisa Jean Moore in 1998: "the 'new and improved' bodily product that semen banks advertise to clients through their informational pamphlets. Technosemen is the result of technologically based semen analysis and manipulation." It refers to any semen that has been donated, manipulated through washing or other techniques, and then advertised for sale for sperm banks as superior to, or more fertile than, natural semen.

Testicular sperm extraction (TESE) and testicular sperm aspiration (TESA)

The use of specialized needles and surgical instruments to extract sperm directly from the testicles for IVF, conducted under anesthetic on men who have sperm production problems, a previous vasectomy, or blockages in the vas deferens.

Tubal insufflation

A technique for detecting blockages in the fallopian tubes popularized by Isidor C. Rubin starting in 1919. A physician pumps oxygen and carbonic acid gas into the tubal duct, and the resulting pressure measurement indicates the presence or absence of a blockage. If the gas releases into the abdomen and causes shoulder pain, the fallopian tubes are not obstructed.

Vitrification

The ultra-rapid cooling of oocytes and embryos into a glasslike form using one or more cryoprotectants, then placed into a carrier such as an open-pulled straw, an electron microscopy grid, or nylon loop. In the present, eggs and embryos are most often preserved using a Cryotop, a thin strip of transparent film that can withstand immersion in liquid nitrogen.

Zygote intrafallopian transfer (ZIFT)

The process of fertilizing sperm and egg in a petri dish and then implanting the fertilized egg into the fallopian tube, so that the egg will implant in the uterus on its own. This procedure is rarely used in the present, as it has a much lower success rate than IVF, in which the egg is implanted in the uterus.

NOTES

Chapter 1

1. J. Marion Sims, *Clinical Notes on Uterine Surgery: With Special Reference to the Management of the Sterile Condition* (New York: William Wood & Co., 1866), 367.

2. Sims, *Clinical Notes on Uterine Surgery*, 369; Margaret Marsh and Wanda Ronner, *The Empty Cradle: Infertility in America from Colonial Times to the Present* (Baltimore, MD: Johns Hopkins University Press, 1996), 66.

3. Katharine Dow, *Making a Good Life: An Ethnography of Nature, Ethics, and Reproduction* (Princeton, NJ: Princeton University Press, 2016), 188.

4. "Infertility," World Health Organization, September 14, 2020, https://www.who.int/news-room/fact-sheets/detail/infertility; Tracey Monaghan and Gayle Davis, "Introduction: Defining the 'Problem': Perspectives on Infertility," in *Palgrave Handbook of Infertility in History: Approaches, Contexts and Perspectives*, ed. Gayle Davis and Tracey Monaghan (London: Palgrave Macmillan, 2017), 29–35; Sally Bishop Shigley, "Great Expectations: Infertility, Disability, and Possibility," in *Palgrave Handbook of Infertility*, 37–55.

5. Gayle Davis and Tracey Monaghan, "Introduction: Infertility in History; Approaches, Contexts and Perspectives," in *Palgrave Handbook of Infertility*, 1–25, esp. 8.

6. Renate Duelli Klein, "What's 'New' about the 'New' Reproductive Technologies?," in Gena Corea et al., *Man-Made Women: How New Reproductive Technologies Affect Women* (London: Hutchinson, 1985), 64–73, esp. 66.

7. Dow, *Making a Good Life*, 160.

8. Sarah Ferber et al., *IVF and Assisted Reproduction: A Global History* (Singapore: Palgrave Macmillan, 2020), 15.

9. M. James Whitelaw, "Use of the Cervical Cap to Increase Fertility in Cases of Oligospermia," *Fertility and Sterility* 1, no. 1 (January–February 1950): 33–39; Frederick M. Hanson and John Rock, "Artificial Insemination with Husband's Sperm," *Fertility and Sterility* 2, no. 2 (March 1951): 162–174, esp. 168.

10. Virpi Ylänne, "Representations of Ageing and Infertility in the Twenty-First-Century British Press," in *Palgrave Handbook of Infertility*, 509–30, esp. 520–521, 526–527.

11. Sarah Franklin, *Embodied Progress: A Cultural Account of Assisted Conception* (London: Routledge, 1997), 202.

Chapter 2

1. Shurlee Swain, "The Interplay between Infertility and Adoption in Policy and Practice in Twentieth-Century Australia," in *Palgrave Handbook of Infertility*, 415–430, esp. 420.

2. Barbara Orland, "The Invention of Artificial Fertilization in the Eighteenth and Nineteenth Century," *History and Philosophy of the Life Sciences* 39 (2017): article 11; F. N. L. Poynter, "Hunter, Spallanzani, and the History of Artificial Insemination," in *Medicine, Science and Culture: Historical Essays in Honor of Owsei Temkin*, ed. Lloyd G. Stevenson and Robert P. Multhauf (Baltimore, MD: Johns Hopkins University Press, 1968), 97–113; Hermann Rohleder, *Die Zeugung beim Menschen in ihren normalen, pathologischen und künstlichen Formen* [Human procreation in its normal, pathological, and artificial forms] (Leipzig: G. Thieme, 1921).

3. Bridget E. Gurtler, "Synthetic Conception: Artificial Insemination and the Transformation of Reproduction and Family in Nineteenth- and Twentieth-Century America" (PhD diss., Rutgers University, 2013), 44n73.

4. Angus McLaren, *Reproduction by Design: Sex, Robots, Trees, and Test-Tube Babies in Interwar Britain* (Chicago: University of Chicago Press, 2012), 115; Louis Girault, *Etude sur la génération artificielle dans l'espèce humaine lue à la Société médicale du Panthéon* [Study on artificial generation in the human species read at the Panthéon Medical Society] (Paris: Aux Bureaux de l'Abeille Medicale, 1869).

5. J. Marion Sims, *On the Treatment of Vesico-Vaginal Fistula* (Philadelphia: Blanchard & Lea, 1853); Deirdre Cooper Owens, *Medical Bondage: Race, Gender, and the Origins of American Gynecology* (Athens: University of Georgia Press, 2018), 80.

6. Margaret Marsh and Wanda Ronner, *The Empty Cradle: Infertility in America from Colonial Times to the Present* (Baltimore, MD: Johns Hopkins University Press, 1996), 73; see also Elaine Tyler May, *Barren in the Promised Land: Childless Americans and the Pursuit of Happiness* (Cambridge, MA: Harvard University Press, 1997), 43–44; and Gurtler, "Synthetic Conception," 59.

7. Owens, *Medical Bondage*, 97.

8. Shannon Withycombe, *Lost: Miscarriage in Nineteenth-Century America* (New Brunswick, NJ: Rutgers University Press, 2018).

9. For example, there were three German editions of J. Marion Sims, *J. Marion Sims's Klinik der Gebärmutter-Chirurgie mit besonderer Berücksichtigung der Behandlung der Sterilität* [J. Marion Sims's uterine surgery clinic with special attention to the treatment of sterility], trans. Hermann Beigel (Erlangen, Germany: Enke, 1866). See also J. Marion Sims, *Notes cliniques sur la chirurgie*

utérine dans ses rapports avec le traitement de la stérilité [Clinical notes on uterine surgery with reports on the treatment of sterility], trans. Dr. Lheritier (Paris: Victor Masson et fils, 1866).

10. Naomi Pfeffer, *The Stork and the Syringe: A Political History of Reproductive Medicine* (Cambridge: Polity Press, 1993), 39, 55; Gurtler, "Synthetic Conception," 22; J. Marion Sims, "Illustrations of the Value of the Microscope in the Treatment of the Sterile Condition," *British Medical Journal* 2 (1868): 465–466, 492–494; Max Huhner, *Sterility in the Male and Female and Its Treatment* (New York: Rebman, 1913).

11. Bridget Gurtler, "From 'Fructification' to 'Insemination': Nomenclature and the Practice of Artificial Insemination," in *Palgrave Handbook of Infertility in History: Approaches, Contexts and Perspectives*, ed. Gayle Davis and Tracey Monaghan (London: Palgrave Macmillan, 2017), 77–98, esp. 80–82; Gurtler, "Synthetic Conception," 61; Edward Bliss Foote, *Plain Home Talk about the Human System* (New York: Murray Hill, 1870); Caroline Rusterholz, *Women's Medicine: Sex, Family Planning and British Female Doctors in Transnational Perspective, 1920–1970* (Manchester: Manchester University Press, 2020), 126; "Any Questions?," *British Medical Journal*, January 29, 1955, https://www.bmj.com/content/1/4908/301; Marsh and Ronner, *Empty Cradle*, 69.

12. Gurtler, "Synthetic Conception," 46, 53.

13. Gurtler, "From 'Fructification' to 'Insemination,'" 82–84; Gurtler, "Synthetic Conception," 52; Michael Finn, "Female Sterilization and Artificial Insemination at the French Fin de Siècle: Facts and Fictions," *Journal of the History of Sexuality* 18, no. 1 (January 2009): 26–43; Joseph Gérard, *Nouvelles causes de stérilité dans les deux sexes: Fécondation artificielle comme moyen ultime de traitement* [Causes and treatment of sterility in both sexes: Fecundation by artificial methods] (Paris: C. Marpon and E. Flammarion, 1888).

14. Fabrice Cahen, "Obstacles to the Establishment of a Policy to Combat Infertility in France, 1920–1950," in *Palgrave Handbook of Infertility*, ed. Davis and Monaghan, 199–219, esp. 207; Alan F. Guttmacher, "Artificial Insemination," *DePaul Law Review* 18, nos. 2–3 (Summer 1969): 566–583, esp. 578.

15. A. D. Hard, "Artificial Impregnation," *Medical World* 27 (April 1909): 163–164; A. T. Gregoire and Robert C. Mayer, "The Impregnators," *Fertility and Sterility* 16, no. 1 (January–February 1965): 130–134. See also May, *Barren in the Promised Land*, 65–69; and Laura Mamo, *Queering Reproduction: Achieving Pregnancy in the Age of Technoscience* (Durham, NC: Duke University Press, 2007), 26–27.

16. Kara W. Swanson, *Banking on the Body: The Market in Blood, Milk, and Sperm in Modern America* (Cambridge, MA: Harvard University Press, 2014),

201; Eliza M. Mosher, "Instrumental Impregnation," *Woman's Medical Journal* 22 (October 1912): 224–225; Robert L. Dickinson, "Artificial Impregnation: Essays in Tubal Insemination," *Transactions of the American Gynecological Society* 45 (1920): 141–148; Robert L. Dickinson, "Suggestions for a Program for American Gynecology," *Transactions of the American Gynecological Society* 45 (1920): 6–7; Andrea Hommel, "Hermann Rohleder (1866–1934) und die Anfänge der künstlichen Befructung in Deutschland [Hermann Rohleder (1866–1934) and the beginnings of artificial insemination in Germany]," *Medizinhistorisches Journal* 29, no. 2 (1994): 121–148, esp. 138–141.

17. Frank P. Davis, *Impotency, Sterility, and Artificial Impregnation* (St. Louis: C. V. Mosby Co., 1917), 106.

18. Theodoor H. van de Velde, *Fertility and Sterility in Marriage: Their Voluntary Promotion and Limitation*, trans. F. W. Stella Browne (1929; London: William Heinemann [Medical Books] Ltd., 1934), 263. For nearly identical descriptions of this process by US physicians, see Mosher, "Instrumental Impregnation," 224–225, and Samuel R. Meaker, "Some Aspects of the Problem of Sterility," *Boston Medical and Surgical Journal* 187, no. 15 (October 12, 1922): 535–539. Dickinson also suggested the use of a test tube for sperm collection in Dickinson, "Artificial Impregnation," 141–148.

19. Van de Velde, *Fertility and Sterility in Marriage*, 266.

20. Van de Velde, *Fertility and Sterility in Marriage*, 207–208; Max Nassauer, "Zur Frage der künstlichen Befruchtung: Fructulet, ein neues Verfahren zur instrumentellen Behandlung der weiblichen Sterilitat [On the question of artificial insemination: Fructulet, a new method for the mechanical treatment of female sterility]," *Münchener medizinische Wochenschrift* 67 (1920): 1463–1465; Hommel, "Hermann Rohleder (1866–1934)," 136.

21. Van de Velde, *Fertility and Sterility in Marriage*, 218.

22. Anne Hanley, "'The Great Foe to the Reproduction of the Race': Diagnosing and Treating Infertility Caused by Venereal Diseases, 1880–1914," in *Palgrave Handbook of Infertility*, ed. Davis and Monaghan, 335–358.

23. Marsh and Ronner, *Empty Cradle*, 150; Margaret Marsh and Wanda Ronner, *The Fertility Doctor: John Rock and the Reproductive Revolution* (Baltimore, MD: Johns Hopkins University Press, 2008), 64; Pfeffer, *Stork and the Syringe*, 125.

24. Lisa Jean Moore, *Sperm Counts: Overcome by Man's Most Precious Fluid* (New York: New York University Press, 2007), 26; D. Macomber and M. Sanders, "The Spermatozoa Count: Its Value in the Diagnosis, Prognosis, and Treatment of Sterility," *New England Journal of Medicine* 200, no. 19 (1929): 981–984; Gerald L. Moench, "Sperm Morphology in Relation to Fertility,"

American Journal of Obstetrics and Gynecology 22, no. 2 (August 1931): 199–210; Gerald L. Moench and Helen Holt, "Microdissection Studies on Human Spermatozoa," *Biological Bulletin* 56, no. 4 (1929): 267–273; Charis Thompson, *Making Parents: The Ontological Choreography of Reproductive Technologies* (Cambridge, MA: MIT Press, 2005), 123.

25. Sandra P. González-Santos, *A Portrait of Assisted Reproduction in Mexico: Scientific, Political, and Cultural Interactions* (Cham: Palgrave Macmillan, 2020), 52–54.

26. C. Travers Stepita, "Physiologic Artificial Insemination," *American Journal of Surgery* 21, no. 3 (September 1933): 450–451.

27. Gurtler, "Synthetic Conception," 220; Frederick M. Hanson and John Rock, "Artificial Insemination with Husband's Sperm," *Fertility and Sterility* 2, no. 2 (March 1951): 162–174, esp. 165; Edmond J. Farris, *Human Fertility and Problems of the Male* (New York: The Author's Press, 1950), 160–161; Sheldon Payne and Robert F. Skeels, "Fertility as Evaluated by Artificial Insemination," *Fertility and Sterility* 5, no. 1 (January 1954): 32–39, esp. 38.

28. Pfeffer, *Stork and the Syringe*, 144; Marsh and Ronner, *Fertility Doctor*, 68.

29. Marsh and Ronner, *Empty Cradle*, 159; Marsh and Ronner, *Fertility Doctor*, 120, 327n14; Meaker, *Human Sterility*, 240–45.

30. Van de Velde, *Fertility and Sterility in Marriage*, 202, 203.

31. Marsh and Ronner, *Empty Cradle*, 175, 191; Pfeffer, *Stork and the Syringe*, 66.

32. William L. Estes, "A Method of Implanting Ovarian Tissue in Order to Maintain Ovarian Function," *Pennsylvania Medical Journal* 13 (May 1910): 610–613, esp. 611; W. L. Estes, Jr., "Ovarian Implantation: The Preservation of Ovarian Function after Operation for Disease of the Pelvic Viscera," *Surgery, Gynecology and Obstetrics* 38 (1924): 394–398; C. E. Adams, "Consequences of Accelerated Ovum Transport, Including a Re-Evaluation of Estes' Operation," *Journal of Reproduction and Fertility* 55, no. 1 (1979): 239–246; Leonard B. Greentree, "The Estes Operation. One Possible Alternative to a 'Test Tube' Baby," *Fertility and Sterility* 32, no. 1 (July 1979): 130–132.

33. Pfeffer, *Stork and the Syringe*, 62–63; Rusterholz, *Women's Medicine*, 120; I. C. Rubin, "Röntgendiagnostik der Uterustumoren mit Hilfe von intrauterinen Collargolinjektionen [X-ray diagnosis of uterine tumors with the help of intrauterine Collargol injections]," *Zentralblatt für Gynäkologie* 18 (May 1914): 658; I. C. Rubin, "Diagnostic Use of Intra-Uterine Iodized Oil Combined with the X-Rays, as Compared to Peruterine CO_2 Insufflation: A Study Based on 66 Cases of Tubal Obstruction," *Radiology* 11, no. 2 (August 1928): 115–125, esp. 115, 122. Le Lorier presented his work at an academic conference but

did not publish it in an academic journal, so it did not have the same reach as Rubin's did.

34. Pfeffer, *Stork and the Syringe*, 64, 135; Marsh and Ronner, *Empty Cradle*, 145; Rubin, "Diagnostic Use of Intra-Uterine Iodized Oil," 122.

35. Van de Velde, *Fertility and Sterility in Marriage*, 218. On the introduction of tubal insufflation to France, see Cahen, "Obstacles to the Establishment," 207.

36. Marsh and Ronner, *Empty Cradle*, 198; Albert Decker and Thomas H. Cherry, "Culdoscopy: A New Method in the Diagnosis of Pelvic Disease— Preliminary Report," *American Journal of Surgery* 64, no. 1 (April 1944): 40–44; González-Santos, *Portrait of Assisted Reproduction in Mexico*, 81.

37. Theodoor H. van de Velde, *Über den Zusammenhang zwischen Ovarial-funktion, Wellenbewegung und Menstrualblutung und über die Entstehung des sogenannten Mittelschmerzes* [On the connection between ovarian function, undulation, and menstrual bleeding and about the development of so-called menstrual pain] (Jena: G. Fisher, 1905); O. L. Harvey and Hazel E. Crockett, "Individual Differences in Temperature Changes of Women during the Course of the Menstrual Cycle," *Human Biology* 4, no. 4 (December 1932): 453–468, esp. 453–454.

38. Anthony Zimmerman, "How Ogino Discovered Rhythm," *The Linacre Quarterly* 62, no. 1 (1995): 29–32; Kyusaku Ogino, "Ovulationstermin und Konzeptionstermin [The ovulation date and the conception date]," *Zentralblatt für Gynäkologie* 54, no. 8 (1930): 464–479; Kyusaku Ogino, *Conception Period of Women*, trans. Yonez Miyagawa (Harrisburg, PA: Medical Arts Publishing Co., 1934).

39. "Österreichische Medizingeschichte: Vor 50 Jahren starb Hermann Knaus [Austrian medical history: Hermann Knaus died fifty years ago]," *Gyn-Activ*, last modified December 14, 2020, https://www.medmedia.at/gyn-aktiv /oesterreichische-medizingeschichte-vor-50-jahren-starb-hermann-knaus/; Hermann Knaus, "Über den Zeitpunkt der Konzeptionsfähigkeit des Weibes [On the timing of women's ability to conceive]," *Archiv für Gynäkologie* 146 (1931): 343–357; Hermann Knaus, *Periodic Fertilty and Sterility in Woman: A Natural Method of Birth Control*, trans. D. H. Kitchin and Kathleen Kitchin (Vienna: Wilhelm Maudrich, 1934); Susanne Krejsa MacManus and Christian Fiala, *Der Detektiv der fruchtbaren Tage: Die Geschichte des Gynäkologen Hermann Knaus* (1892–1970) [The fertile-days detective: The history of the gynecologist Hermann Knaus (1892–1970)] (Vienna: Verlagshaus der Ärzte, 2017).

40. Kyusaku Ogino, "Über den Konzeptionstermin des Weibes und seine Anwendung in der Praxis [On the conception date of women and its application in

practice]," *Zentralblatt für Gynäkologie* 56 (1932): 721–732; Hermann Knaus, "Die Periodische Frucht- und Unfruchtbarkeit des Weibes [The periodic fertility and infertility of women]," *Zentralblatt für Gynäkologie* 57 (1933): 1393–1408; Elisabeth Raith-Paula and Petra Frank-Herrmann, *Natürliche Familienplanung heute: Modernes Zykluswissen für Beratung und Anwendung* [Natural family planning today: Modern cycle knowledge for advice and application], 6th ed. (Berlin: Springer, 2020), 7–14.

41. J. N. J. Smulders, *Periodieke Onthouding in het Huwelijk: Methode Ogino-Knaus* [On periodic abstinence within marriage: The Ogino-Knaus method] (Nijmegen-Utrecht: Decker, van de Vegt en van Leeuwen, 1930); Leo John Latz, *The Rhythm of Sterility and Fertility in Women*, 4th ed. (Chicago: Latz Foundation, 1934); Wannes Dupont, "The Case for Contraception: Medicine, Morality, and Sexology at the Catholic University of Leuven (1930–1968)," *Histoire, Médicine, et Santé* 13 (Summer 2018): 49–65; Pfeffer, *Stork and the Syringe*, 131.

42. Jenna Caitlin Healey, "Sooner or Later: Age, Pregnancy, and the Reproductive Revolution in Late Twentieth-Century America" (PhD diss., Yale University, 2016), 243–247, esp. 243, 246; Joseph B. Doyle, "Cervical Tampon Synchronous Test for Ovulation: Simultaneous Assay of Glucose from Cervix and Follicular Fluid from Cul-de-Sac and Ovary by Culdotomy," *Journal of the American Medical Association* 167, no. 12 (July 19, 1958): 1464–1469; Joseph B. Doyle, Frank J. Ewers, Jr., and Donald Sapit, "The New Fertility Testing Tape: A Predictive Test of the Fertile Period," *Journal of the American Medical Association* 172, no. 16 (April 16, 1960): 1744–1750.

43. Pfeffer, *Stork and the Syringe*, 76; Margaret Hadley Jackson et al., "Artificial Insemination (Donor)," *The Eugenics Review* 48, no. 4 (January 1957): 203–211; Marsh and Ronner, *Empty Cradle*, 163; González-Santos, *Portrait of Assisted Reproduction in Mexico*, 51, 55, 99; Daphna Birenbaum-Carmeli, "Thirty-Five Years of Assisted Reproductive Technologies in Israel," *Reproductive BioMedicine and Society Online* 2 (June 2016): 16–23; Chia-Ling Wu, "Managing Multiple Masculinities in Donor Insemination: Doctors Configuring Infertile Men and Sperm Donors in Taiwan," *Sociology of Health & Illness* 33, no. 1 (January 2011): 96–113, esp. 101; Kara W. Swanson, "Adultery by Doctor: Artificial Insemination, 1890–1945," *Chicago-Kent Law Review* 87, no. 2 (April 2012): 591–633, esp. 603.

44. Dickinson, "Artificial Impregnation," 144; Swanson, *Banking on the Body*, 207, 208; Sophia J. Kleegman, "Practical and Ethical Aspects of Artificial Insemination," *Advances in Sex Research* 1 (October 1963): 112–118, esp. 114–115.

45. Guttmacher, "Artificial Insemination," 572, 574; Swanson, "Adultery by Doctor," 612–613.

46. Swanson, "The Birth of the Sperm Bank," *Annals of Iowa* 71 (Summer 2012): 241–276, esp. 256–257; Gurtler, "Synthetic Conception," 222–26.

47. Gurtler, "Synthetic Conception," 228, Jerome K. Sherman, "Research on Frozen Sperm," *Fertility and Sterility* 14, no. 1 (January 1963): 49–64.

48. Mamo, *Queering Reproduction*, 29; Kleegman, "Practical and Ethical Aspects of Artificial Insemination," 118; Swanson, *Banking on the Body*, 214.

49. Stine W. Adrian, "Subversive Practices of Sperm Donation: Globalising Danish Sperm," in *Critical Kinship Studies*, ed. Charlotte Kroløkke, Lene Myong, Stine W. Adrian, and Tine Tjørnhøj-Thomsen (London: Rowman and Littlefield, 2016), 185–202, esp. 185; Swanson, *Banking on the Body*, 219; Rene Almeling, *Sex Cells: The Medical Market for Eggs and Sperm* (Berkeley: University of California Press, 2011), 29.

50. Mamo, *Queering Reproduction*, 29; Almeling, *Sex Cells*, 30; Gurtler, "Synthetic Conception," 222–226.

51. Swanson, *Banking on the Body*, 230.

52. Almeling, *Sex Cells*, 29, 57; Charlotte Kroløkke, "Click a Donor: Viking Masculinity on the Line," *Journal of Consumer Culture* 9, no. 1 (March 2009): 7–30, esp. 14; Swanson, *Banking on the Body*, 231; see also Sandra Patton-Imani, *Queering Family Trees: Race, Reproductive Justice, and Lesbian Parenthood* (New York: New York University Press, 2020), 90.

53. Stine W. Adrian, "Rethinking Reproductive Selection: Traveling Transnationally for Sperm," *BioSocieties* 15, no. 4 (December 2020): 532–554, esp. 537; Moore, *Sperm Counts*, 101.

54. Ayo Wahlberg, *Good Quality: The Routinization of Sperm Banking in China* (Oakland: University of California Press, 2018), 38, 46, 25.

55. Wahlberg, *Good Quality*, 109.

56. Wahlberg, *Good Quality*, 134.

57. Wahlberg, *Good Quality*, 109, 179.

Chapter 3

1. Leopold Schenk, "Das Säugethierei künstlich befruchtet außerhalb des Mutterleibes [The mammalian egg artificially fertilized outside the womb]," *Mitteilungen des Embryologischen Institutes der K.K. Universität Wien*, 1 (1878): 107; Margaret Marsh and Wanda Ronner, *The Pursuit of Parenthood: Reproductive Technology from Test-Tube Babies to Uterus Implants* (Baltimore, MD: Johns Hopkins University Press, 2019), 18–19; William Clifford Roberts, "Facts and

Ideas from Anywhere," *Baylor University Medical Center Proceedings* 28, no. 3 (July 2015): 421–432, esp. 424–425.

2. Roberts, "Facts and Ideas from Anywhere," 427; Margaret Marsh and Wanda Ronner, *The Fertility Doctor: John Rock and the Reproductive Revolution* (Baltimore, MD: Johns Hopkins University Press, 2008), 51.

3. Marsh and Ronner, *Fertility Doctor*, 90–99; Marsh and Ronner, *Pursuit of Parenthood*, 17; Arthur T. Hertig, "A Fifteen-Year Search for First-Stage Human Ova," *Journal of the American Medical Association* 261, no. 3 (January 20, 1989): 434–435; A. T. Hertig and J. Rock, "Searching for Early Fertilized Human Ova," *Gynecologic Investigation* 4 (1973): 112–139; A. T. Hertig and J. Rock, "Two Human Ova of the Pre-Villous Stage, Having an Ovulation Age of about Eleven and Twelve Days Respectively," *Contributions to Embryology* 29 (1941): 127–156; A. T. Hertig and J. Rock, "Two Human Ova of the Pre-Villous Stage, Having a Developmental Age of about Seven and Nine Days, Respectively," *Contributions to Embryology* 33 (1945): 65–84.

4. Marsh and Ronner, *Fertility Doctor*, 106–110; Marsh and Ronner, *Pursuit of Parenthood*, 21–22; Margaret Marsh, "Americans and Assisted Reproduction: The Past as Prologue," in *Palgrave Handbook of Infertility in History: Approaches, Contexts and Perspectives*, ed. Gayle Davis and Tracey Monaghan (London: Palgrave Macmillan, 2017), 545–64, esp. 548–551; John Rock and Miriam Menkin, "In Vitro Fertilization and Cleavage of Human Ovarian Eggs," *Science* 100, no. 2588 (August 4, 1944): 105–107; Miriam Menkin and John Rock, "In Vitro Fertilization and Cleavage of Human Ovarian Eggs," *American Journal of Obstetrics & Gynecology* 55, no. 3 (March 1948): 440–451.

5. Shlomo Mashiach et al., "The Contribution of Israeli Researchers to Reproductive Medicine," in *Kin, Gene, Community: Reproductive Technologies among Jewish Israelis*, ed. Daphna Birenbaum-Carmeli and Yoram S. Carmeli (New York: Berghahn Books, 2010), 51–60. See also Laura Mamo, *Queering Reproduction: Achieving Pregnancy in the Age of Technoscience* (Durham, NC: Duke University Press, 2007), 28.

6. Patrick Steptoe and Robert Edwards, *A Matter of Life: The Story of a Medical Breakthrough* (London: Sphere Books, 1981), 74, 79; John Leeton, *Test Tube Revolution: The Early History of IVF* (Clayton: Monash University Publishing, 2013), 5; Sarah Ferber et al., *IVF and Assisted Reproduction: A Global History* (Singapore: Palgrave Macmillan, 2020), 33.

7. Catherine Waldby, *The Oocyte Economy: The Changing Meaning of Human Eggs* (Durham, NC: Duke University Press, 2019), 59; Leeton, *Test Tube Revolution*, 11; Jacques Cohen, "The Track to Assisted Reproduction: From Animal to

Human In-Vitro Fertilization," in *In-Vitro Fertilization: The Pioneers' History*, ed. Gabor Kovacs, Peter Brinsden, and Alan DeCherney (Cambridge: Cambridge University Press, 2018), 8–20, esp. 9; Robert Chambers, "New Micromanipulator and Methods for the Isolation of a Single Bacterium and the Manipulation of Living Cells," *Journal of Infectious Diseases* 31, no. 4 (October 1922): 334–343.

8. Cohen, "Track to Assisted Reproduction," 14.

9. Steptoe and Edwards, *Matter of Life*, 80, 82; Waldby, *Oocyte Economy*, 59; Ferber et al., *IVF and Assisted Reproduction*, 36; Sarah Franklin, *Biological Relatives: IVF, Stem Cells, and the Future of Kinship* (Durham, NC: Duke University Press, 2013), 106.

10. Ferber et al., *IVF and Assisted Reproduction*, 35–37; Cohen, "Track to Assisted Reproduction," 13.

11. Jean Cohen et al., "The Early Days of IVF Outside the UK," *Human Reproduction Update* 11, no. 5 (September–October 2005): 439–460; Marsh and Ronner, *Pursuit of Parenthood*, 40, 62.

12. Cohen, "Track to Assisted Reproduction," 15.

13. Leeton, *Test Tube Revolution*, 31; Cohen et al., "Early Days of IVF Outside the UK," 443; Peter Renou et al., "The Collection of Human Oocytes for In Vitro Fertilization: An Instrument for Maximizing Oocyte Recovery Rate," *Fertility and Sterility* 35, no. 4 (April 1981): 409–412; Marsh, "Americans and Assisted Reproduction," 556.

14. Judith Lasker and Susan Borg, *In Search of Parenthood* (Philadelphia: Temple University Press, 1994), 50; Sandra P. González-Santos, *A Portrait of Assisted Reproduction in Mexico: Scientific, Political, and Cultural Interactions* (Cham: Palgrave Macmillan, 2020), 101.

15. González-Santos, *Portrait of Assisted Reproduction in Mexico*, 179.

16. González-Santos, *Portrait of Assisted Reproduction in Mexico*, 181; Cohen, "Track to Assisted Reproduction," 17.

17. Charis Thompson, *Making Parents: The Ontological Choreography of Reproductive Technologies* (Cambridge, MA: MIT Press, 2005), 197.

18. Waldby, *Oocyte Economy*, 154–155, 70.

19. On the creation of these catheters, see Ferber et al., *IVF and Assisted Reproduction*, 88, and John Lui Yovich and Ian Logan Craft, "Founding Pioneers of IVF: Independent Innovative Researchers Generating Livebirths within 4 Years of the First Birth," *Reproductive Biology* 18 (2018): 317–323, esp. 320, 321; Christine Crowe, "Whose Mind over Whose Matter? Women, In Vitro Fertilization, and the Development of Scientific Knowledge," in *The New Reproductive Technologies,* ed. Maureen McNeil, Ian Varcoe, and Steven Yearley (Houndmills: Macmillan Press, 1990), 27–57, esp. 31.

20. Sarah Franklin, *Embodied Progress: A Cultural Account of Assisted Conception* (London: Routledge, 1997), 108–109; Marsh and Ronner, *Pursuit of Parenthood*, 3.

21. Lasker and Borg, *In Search of Parenthood*, 67; Thompson, *Making Parents*, 96–98.

22. Diane Tober, *Romancing the Sperm: Shifting Biopolitics and the Making of Modern Families* (New Brunswick, NJ: Rutgers University Press, 2018), 72; Manuela Perrotta and Josie Hamper, "The Crafting of Hope. Contextualizing Add-Ons in the Treatment Trajectories of IVF Patients," *Social Science & Medicine* 287, no. 114317 (2021): 1–8.

23. Marsh and Ronner, *Pursuit of Parenthood*, 89, 122–126; González-Santos, *Portrait of Assisted Reproduction in Mexico*, 130, 147; Mary Dodge and Gilbert Geis, *Stealing Dreams: A Fertility Clinic Scandal* (Boston: Northeastern University Press, 2003).

24. J. L. Yovich et al., "Pregnancies Following Pronuclear Stage Tubal Transfer," *Fertility and Sterility* 48, no. 5 (November 1987): 851–857; Thomas B. Pool et al., "Zygote Intrafallopian Transfer as a Treatment for Nontubal Infertility: A 2-Year Study," *Fertility and Sterility* 54, no. 3 (September 1990): 482–488; C. Matthew Peterson et al., "Ovulation Induction with Gonadotropins and Intrauterine Insemination Compared with In Vitro Fertilization and No Therapy: A Prospective, Nonrandomized, Cohort Study and Meta-Analysis," *Fertility and Sterility* 62, no. 3 (September 1994): 535–544.

25. André Van Steirteghem, "The Brussels Story and the Eureka Moment of Intracytoplasmic Sperm Injection," in *In-Vitro Fertilization*, ed. Kovacs et al., 84–86, esp. 84, 85.

26. Sarah Franklin, "Embryo Watching: How IVF Has Remade Biology," *Technoscienza* 4, no. 1 (June 2013): 23–43, esp. 35.

27. Susan Martha Kahn, "The Mirth of the Clinic: Field Notes from an Israeli Fertility Center," in *Kin, Gene, Community*, ed. Birenbaum-Carmeli and Carmeli, 206–317, esp. 300.

28. Cohen, "Track to Assisted Reproduction," 14; Rene Almeling, *Sex Cells: The Medical Market for Eggs and Sperm* (Berkeley: University of California Press, 2011), 33; Thompson, *Making Parents*, 124.

29. Ayo Wahlberg and Tine M. Gammeltoft, "Introduction: Kinds of Children," in *Selective Reproduction in the 21st Century*, ed. Ayo Wahlberg and Tine M. Gammeltoft (Cham: Palgrave Macmillan, 2017), 1–25, esp. 6.

30. Toni Weschler, *Taking Charge of Your Fertility: The Definitive Guide to Natural Birth Control, Pregnancy Achievement, and Reproductive Health*, 20th anniversary ed. (New York: HarperCollins, 2015), 250.

31. Vincenzo Pavone and Sara Lafuente Funes, "Selecting What? Pre-Implantation Genetic Diagnosis and Screening Trajectories in Spain," in *Selective Reproduction in the 21st Century*, ed. Wahlberg and Gammeltoft, 123–148, esp. 130, 141.

32. Junhao Yan et al., "Live Birth with or without Preimplantation Genetic Testing for Aneuploidy," *New England Journal of Medicine* 385, no. 22 (November 25, 2021): 2047–2058.

33. Ferber et al., *IVF and Assisted Reproduction*, 37, 52–53; Aditya Bharadwaj, "The Indian IVF Saga: A Contested History," *Reproductive BioMedicine and Society Online* 2 (June 2016): 54–61, esp. 55–56.

34. Waldby, *Oocyte Economy*, 62, 75; Ferber et al., *IVF and Assisted Reproduction*, 74.

35. Ferber et al., *IVF and Assisted Reproduction*, 88, 160, 161; Gena Corea, *The Mother Machine: Reproductive Technologies from Artificial Insemination to Artificial Wombs* (New York: Harper & Row, 1985), 87–88.

36. Marsh and Ronner, *Pursuit of Parenthood*, 90, 95; Thompson, *Making Parents*, 194.

37. Marsh and Ronner, *Empty Cradle*, 248; Leeton, *Test Tube Revolution*, 1, 49; Andrea Whittaker, "From 'Mung Ming' to 'Baby Gammy': A Local History of Assisted Reproduction in Thailand," *Reproductive BioMedicine and Society Online* 2 (June 2016): 71–78, esp. 73.

38. Thompson, *Making Parents*, 197; Almeling, *Sex Cells*, 91, 92; Ferber et al., *IVF and Assisted Reproduction*, 35–37.

39. Debra A. Gook, "History of Oocyte Preservation," *Reproductive BioMedicine Online* 23, no. 3 (September 2011): 281–289, esp. 282–283.

40. Anna Molas and Andrea Whittaker, "Beyond the Making of Altruism: Branding and Identity in Egg Donation Websites in Spain," *BioSocieties* 17 (2021): 320–346, esp. 338, 339.

41. Diane Tober and Charlotte Kroløkke, "Emotion, Embodiment, and Reproductive Colonialism in the Global Human Egg Trade," *Gender, Work, and Organization* 28, no. 5 (September 2021): 1766–1786, esp. 1774; Amrita Pande and Tessa Moll, "Gendered Bio-Responsibilities and Travelling Egg Providers from South Africa," *Reproductive Biomedicine and Society Online* 6 (August 2018): 23–33, esp. 29.

42. Pande and Moll, "Gendered Bio-Responsibilities," 27; Amrita Pande, "Visa Stamps for Injections: Traveling Biolabor and South African Egg Provision," *Gender & Society* 34, no. 4 (August 2020): 573–596, esp. 576, 577.

43. Waldby, *Oocyte Economy*, 6; Almeling, *Sex Cells*, 76. See also Margaret Boulos, Ian Kerridge, and Catherine Waldby, "Reciprocity in the Donation of

Reproductive Oöcytes," in *Reframing Reproduction: Conceiving Gendered Experiences*, ed. Meredith Nash (Houndmills: Palgrave Macmillan, 2014), 203–220.

44. Lucy van de Wiel, *Freezing Fertility: Oocyte Cryopreservation and the Gender Politics of Aging* (New York: New York University Press, 2020), 3.

45. Waldby, *Oocyte Economy*, 122; Van de Wiel, *Freezing Fertility*, 6; K. Paul Katayama et al., "High Survival Rate of Vitrified Human Oocytes Results in Clinical Pregnancy," *Fertility and Sterility* 80, no. 1 (July 2003): 223–224; Gook, "History of Oocyte Preservation," 285.

46. Catherine Waldby, "'Banking Time': Egg Freezing and the Negotiation of Future Fertility," *Culture, Health, & Sexuality* 17, no. 4 (2015): 470–482, esp. 472.

47. "Vitrification: Cryotop®," Kitazato, accessed April 24, 2022, https://www.kitazato-ivf.com/vitrification/cryotop; O. Bern et al., "Successful Vitrification of Human Embryos Using Equilibration Solution," *Fertility and Sterility* 106, no. 3, supplement (September 2016): e139; Shingo Mitsuhata et al., "Effect of Equilibration Time on Clinical and Neonatal Outcomes in Human Blastocysts Vitrification," *Reproductive Medicine and Biology* 19, no. 3 (July 2020): 270–276.

48. Waldby, *Oocyte Economy*, 120.

49. Daphna Birenbaum-Carmeli, Marcia C. Inhorn, Mira D. Vale, and Pasquale Patrizio, "Cryopreserving Jewish Motherhood: Egg Freezing in Israel and the United States," *Medical Anthropology Quarterly* 35, no. 3 (September 2021): 346–63, esp. 351, 356; Zeynep B. Gürtin and Emily Tiemann, "The Marketing of Elective Egg Freezing: A Content, Cost, and Quality Analysis of UK Fertility Clinic Websites," *Reproductive BioMedicine Online* 12 (March 2021): 56–68, esp. 61; Laura Briggs, *How All Politics Became Reproductive Politics: From Welfare Reform to Foreclosure to Trump* (Oakland: University of California Press, 2017), 107–116.

50. Jenna Caitlin Healey, "Sooner or Later: Age, Pregnancy, and the Reproductive Revolution in Late Twentieth-Century America" (PhD diss., Yale University, 2016), 18.

51. Kylie Baldwin, *Egg Freezing, Fertility and Reproductive Choice: Negotiating Responsibility, Hope, and Modern Motherhood* (Bingley: Emerald Press, 2019), 13; Kylie Baldwin, "The Biomedicalization of Reproductive Ageing: Reproductive Citizenship and the Gendering of Fertility Risk," *Health, Risk, & Society* 21, nos. 5–6 (2019): 268–283, esp. 272; see also Lauren Jade Martin, "Anticipating Infertility: Egg Freezing, Genetic Preservation, and Risk," *Gender and Society*, 24, no. 4 (2010): 526–545.

52. Waldby, *Oocyte Economy*, 127, 128.

53. Waldby, *Oocyte Economy*, 126, 133.

54. Van de Wiel, *Freezing Fertility*, 95, 110; see also Thompson, *Making Parents*, 10.

55. Waldby, *Oocyte Economy*, 134 (emphasis in original), 135; see also Van de Wiel, *Freezing Fertility*, 183; and Stine W. Adrian, "Subversive Practices of Sperm Donation: Globalising Danish Sperm," in *Critical Kinship Studies*, ed. Charlotte Kroløkke, Lene Myong, Stine W. Adrian, and Tine Tjørnhøj-Thomsen (London: Rowman and Littlefield, 2016), 188.

56. Maria Elisabetta Coccia et al., "'Two Countries-Two Labs': The Transnational Gamete Donation (TGD) Programme to Support Egg Donation," *Journal of Assisted Reproduction and Genetics* 37 (2020): 3039–3049; Wahlberg and Gammeltoft, "Introduction: Kinds of Children," 7.

57. Waldby, *Oocyte Economy*, 67; "Older Women Exploited by IVF Clinics, Says Fertility Watchdog," *BBC News*, last modified April 22, 2019, https://www.bbc.com/news/uk-48008635; "Fertility Treatment 2019: Trends and Figures," Human Fertilisation and Embryology Authority, last modified May 2021, https://www.hfea.gov.uk/about-us/publications/research-and-data/fertility-treatment-2019-trends-and-figures.

58. Fernando Zegers-Hochschild et al., "Celebrating 30 Years of ART in Latin America; and the 2018 Report," *Reproductive BioMedicine Online* 43, no. 3 (September 2021): 475–490, esp. 481, 484.

59. Giulia Cavaliere and James Rupert Fletcher, "Age-Discriminated IVF Access and Evidence-Based Ageism: Is There a Better Way?," *Science, Technology, & Human Values* (2021): preprint, 1–25.

60. Pfeffer, *Stork and the Syringe*, 164.

61. Franklin, *Biological Relatives*, 35.

Chapter 4

1. Amrita Pande and Tessa Moll, "Gendered Bio-Responsibilities and Travelling Egg Providers from South Africa," *Reproductive Biomedicine and Society Online* 6 (August 2018): 23–33, esp. 24.

2. Stine W. Adrian and Charlotte Kroløkke, "Passport to Parenthood: Reproductive Pathways in and out of Denmark," *NORA—Nordic Journal of Feminist and Gender Research* 26, no. 2 (2018): 112–126, esp. 123–124; Marcia C. Inhorn et al., "Third-Party Reproduction Assistance around the Mediterranean: Comparing Sunni Egypt, Catholic Italy, and Multisectarian Lebanon," in *Islam and Assisted Reproductive Technologies: Sunni and Shia Perspectives*, ed. Marcia C. Inhorn and Soraya Tremayne (New York: Berghahn Books, 2012), 223–260, esp. 227.

3. Amel Alghrani, *Regulating Assisted Reproductive Technologies: New Horizons* (Cambridge: Cambridge University Press, 2018), 15.

4. Inhorn et al., "Third-Party Reproduction Assistance around the Mediterranean," 242, 243; Marcia C. Inhorn et al., "Assisted Reproduction and Middle East Kinship: A Regional and Religious Comparison," *Reproductive BioMedicine and Society Online* 4 (June 2017): 41–51, esp. 46.

5. Alexandra Gruian, "Ova Provision in Romania: Identity Dynamics and Exclusionary Practices" (PhD diss., University of Leeds, 2018), 9, 13.

6. Gruian, "Ova Provision in Romania," 13.

7. Alghrani, *Regulating Assisted Reproductive Technologies*, 49; Raquel María Fernández et al., "Experience of Preimplantation Genetic Diagnosis with HLA Matching at the University Hospital Virgen del Rocío in Spain: Technical and Clinical Overview," *BioMed Research International* (2014): article ID 560160, esp. 2; Mark Henaghan and Thomas Cleary, "The State in Action: An Insider's View of How the State Regulates the Use of PGD with HLA Tissue-Typing in New Zealand," in *Regulating Pre-Implantation Genetic Diagnosis: A Comparative and Theoretical Analysis*, ed. Sheila A. M. McLean and Sarah Elliston (London: Routledge, 2012), 199–223.

8. Malcolm K. Smith, *Saviour Siblings and the Regulation of Assisted Reproductive Technology: Harm, Ethics, and Law* (London: Routledge, 2015), 2, 3–5; Molly Hendrickson, "17 Years Later, Nash Family Opens Up about Controversial Decision to Save Dying Daughter," last modified November 14, 2017, https://www.thedenverchannel.com/news/local-news/17-years-later-nash-family-opens-up-about-controversial-decision-to-save-dying-daughter; Zachary E. Shapiro, "Savior Siblings in the United States: Ethical Conundrums, Legal and Regulatory Void," *Washington and Lee Journal of Civil Rights and Social Justice* 24, no. 2 (April 2018): 419–461, esp. 460.

9. The ESHRE Task Force on Ethics and Law, "Taskforce 7: Ethical Considerations for the Cryopreservation of Gametes and Reproductive Tissues for Self-Use," *Human Reproduction* 19, no. 2 (February 2004): 460–462; Eleri Williams, "A Storage Solution for Embryos and Gametes?," *BioNews*, last modified October 4, 2021, https://www.bionews.org.uk/page_159563; Anna Hecker, "What Should I Do with My Unused Embryos?," *New York Times*, last modified April 15, 2020, https://www.nytimes.com/2020/04/15/parenting/fertility/ivf-unused-frozen-eggs.html.

10. Jasmine Taylor-Coleman, "The Americans Who 'Adopt' Other People's Embryos," *BBC News*, last modified July 18, 2016, https://www.bbc.com/news/magazine-36450328; Mara Simopoulou et al., "Discarding IVF Embryos: Reporting on Global Practices," *Journal of Assisted Reproduction and*

Genetics 36, no. 12 (December 2019): 2447–2457, esp. 2453. See also Risa Cromer, "Making the Ethnic Embryo: Enacting Race in US Embryo Adoption," *Medical Anthropology* 38, no. 7 (2019): 603–619.

11. Ayo Wahlberg and Tine M. Gammeltoft, "Introduction: Kinds of Children," in *Selective Reproduction in the 21st Century*, ed. Ayo Wahlberg and Tine M. Gammeltoft (Cham: Palgrave Macmillan, 2017), 1–25, esp. 17.

12. Adrian and Krarup, "Passport to Parenthood," 113; Charlotte Kroløkke, "Eggs and Euros: A Feminist Perspective on Reproductive Travel from Denmark to Spain," *International Journal of Feminist Approaches to Bioethics* 7, no. 2 (Fall 2014): 144–163; Charlotte Kroløkke et al., *The Cryopolitics of Reproduction on Ice: A New Scandinavian Ice Age* (Bingley: Emerald Press, 2020), 27; Naina Bajekal, "Why So Many Women Travel to Denmark for Fertility Treatment," *Time*, last modified January 3, 2019, https://time.com/5491636/denmark-ivf-storkklinik-fertility.

13. On Germany, see Katja Köppen, Heike Trappe, and Christian Schmitt, "Who Can Take Advantage of Medically Assisted Reproduction in Germany?," *Reproductive Biomedicine and Society Online* 13 (August 2021): 51–61, esp. 52. Austria has allowed donor eggs since February 2015 only with narrow restrictions. See Erich Griessler and Mariella Hager, "Changing Direction: The Struggle of Regulating Assisted Reproductive Technology in Austria," *Reproductive Biomedicine & Society Online* 3 (December 2016): 68–76. On Switzerland, see Sascha Britsko, "Mehr als 'gewollt': Wie weit gehen Frauen für den Kinderwunsch? Mindestens bis nach Alicante [More than "wanted": How far will women go to have children? At least as far as Alicante]," *Neue Zürcher Zeitung*, February 12, 2021, https://www.nzz.ch/schweiz/mehr-als-gewollt-wie-weit-gehen-frauen-fuer-ihren-kinderwunsch-ld.1582010; on Hungary, see Eva-Maria Knoll, "Reproducing Hungarians: Reflections on Fuzzy Boundaries in Reproductive Border Crossing," in *Reproductive Technologies as Global Form: Ethnographies of Knowledges, Practices, and Transnational Encounters*, ed. Michi Knecht, Maren Klotz, and Stefan Beck (Frankfurt: Campus Verlag, 2012), 255–282, and Judit Takás, "Limiting Queer Reproduction in Hungary," *Journal of International Women's Studies* 20, no. 1 (December 2018): 68–80, esp. 69.

14. Lucy van de Wiel, *Freezing Fertility: Oocyte Cryopreservation and the Gender Politics of Aging* (New York: New York University Press, 2020), 183.

15. Giuseppe Benagiano and Luca Gianaroli, "The New Italian IVF Legislation," *Reproductive BioMedicine Online* 9, no. 2 (2004): 117–125; Irene Riezzo et al., "Italian Law on Medically Assisted Reproduction: Do Women's Autonomy and Health Matter?," *BMC Women's Health* (2016): article 44; Giulia Zanini, "Neither Gametes nor Children: Italian Prospective Parents and the Variable

Meaning of Donor Embryos," *Technoscienza* 4, no. 1 (June 2013): 87–109, esp. 98.

16. Trudie Gerrits, "Assisted Reproductive Technologies in Ghana: Transnational Undertakings, Local Practices, and 'More Affordable' IVF," *Reproductive BioMedicine and Society Online* 2 (June 2016): 32–38, esp. 37.

17. Andrea Whittaker, "From 'Mung Ming' to 'Baby Gammy': A Local History of Assisted Reproduction in Thailand," *Reproductive BioMedicine and Society Online* 2 (June 2016): 71–78, esp. 72; see also Leslie R. Schover, "Cross-Border Surrogacy: The Case of Baby Gammy Highlights the Need for Global Agreement on Protections for All Parties," *Fertility and Sterility* 102, no. 5 (November 2014): 1258–1259.

18. Amrita Pande, "Revisiting Surrogacy in India: Domino Effects of the Ban," *Journal of Gender Studies* 30, no. 4 (2021): 395–405, esp. 396, 402.

19. Adrian and Kr" Kr000000 røkke, "Passport to Parenthood"; Stine W. Adrian, "Rethinking Reproductive Selection: Traveling Transnationally for Sperm," *BioSocieties* 15 (December 2020): 532–554.

20. Gayle Davis and Tracey Loughran, "Introduction: Situating Infertility in Medicine," in *Palgrave Handbook of Infertility in History: Approaches, Contexts and Perspectives*, ed. Gayle Davis and Tracey Monaghan (London: Palgrave Macmillan, 2017), 265–71, esp. 269.

21. Theodoor H. van de Velde, *Fertility and Sterility in Marriage: Their Voluntary Promotion and Limitation*, trans. F. W. Stella Browne (1929; London: William Heinemann [Medical Books] Ltd., 1934), 270; Alan F. Guttmacher, "Artificial Insemination," *DePaul Law Review* 18, nos. 2–3 (Summer 1969): 566–83, esp. 578; Pius XI, *Casti connubii* [On Christian marriage], accessed April 24, 2022, https://www.vatican.va/content/pius-xi/en/encyclicals/documents/hf_p-xi_enc_19301231_casti-connubii.html; Sandra P. González-Santos, *A Portrait of Assisted Reproduction in Mexico: Scientific, Political, and Cultural Interactions* (Cham: Palgrave Macmillan, 2020), 53.

22. "Instruction on Respect for Human Life in Its Origin," Congregation for the Doctrine of the Faith, accessed April 24, 2022, https://www.vatican.va/roman_curia/congregations/cfaith/documents/rc_con_cfaith_doc_19870222_respect-for-human-life_en.html.

23. Inhorn et al., "Third-Party Reproduction Assistance around the Mediterranean," 232; "About NaProTechnology," NaProTechnology, accessed April 24, 2022, https://www.naprotechnology.com/about.

24. González-Santos, *Portrait of Assisted Reproduction in Mexico*, 253, 231.

25. Fernando Zegers-Hochschild, "The Development in In-Vitro Fertilization in Latin America," in *In-Vitro Fertilization: The Pioneers' History*, ed. Gabor

Kovacs, Peter Brinsden, and Alan DeCherney (Cambridge: Cambridge University Press, 2018), 147.

26. Marcia C. Inhorn, "Cosmopolitan Conceptions in Global Dubai? The Emiratization of IVF and Its Consequences," *Reproductive BioMedicine and Society Online* 2 (June 2016): 24–31; Soraya Tremayne and Marcia C. Inhorn, "Introduction: Islam and Assisted Reproductive Technologies," in *Islam and Assisted Reproductive Technologies*, ed. Inhorn and Tremayne, 1–23, esp. 14.

27. Tremayne and Inhorn, "Introduction," 3, 9; Soraya Tremayne, "The 'Down Side' of Gamete Donation: Challenging 'Happy Family' Rhetoric in Iran," in *Islam and Assisted Reproductive Technologies*, ed. Inhorn and Tremayne, 130–156, esp. 134; Farouk Mahmoud, "Controversies in Islamic Evaluation of Assisted Reproductive Technologies," in *Islam and Assisted Reproductive Technologies*, ed. Inhorn and Tremayne, 70–99, esp. 80–81.

28. Susan Martha Kahn, *Reproducing Jews: A Cultural Account of Assisted Conception in Israel* (Durham, NC: Duke University Press, 2000), 166.

29. "Egg Donation," State of Israel Ministry of Health, accessed April 24, 2022, https://www.health.gov.il/English/Topics/fertility/Pages/ovum_donation.aspx; Kahn, *Reproducing Jews*, 2, 38–39; Daphna Birenbaum-Carmeli, "Thirty-Five Years of Assisted Reproductive Technologies in Israel," *Reproductive BioMedicine and Society Online* 2 (June 2016): 16–23, esp. 17.

30. Kahn, *Reproducing Jews*, 4, 41, 50, 62.

31. Kahn, *Reproducing Jews*, 77, 173; see also Daphna Birenbaum-Carmeli and Yoram S. Carmeli, "Introduction: Reproductive Technologies among Jewish Israelis: Setting the Ground," in *Kin, Gene, Community: Reproductive Technologies among Jewish Israelis*, ed. Daphna Birenbaum-Carmeli and Yoram S. Carmeli (New York: Berghahn Books, 2010), 1–50.

32. Kahn, *Reproducing Jews*, 77.

33. Gala Rexer, "Borderlands of Reproduction: Bodies, Borders, and Assisted Reproductive Technologies in Israel/Palestine," *Ethnic and Racial Studies* 44, no. 9 (2021): 154–168, esp. 157, 164–165.

34. Sarah Ferber et al., *IVF and Assisted Reproduction: A Global History* (Singapore: Palgrave Macmillan, 2020), 140.

Chapter 5

1. Sandra P. González-Santos, *A Portrait of Assisted Reproduction in Mexico: Scientific, Political, and Cultural Interactions* (Cham: Palgrave Macmillan, 2020), 10.

2. Jil Clark, "Sperm Bank Welcomes Unmarried Recipients," *Gay Community News*, October 30, 1982: 3, quoted in Bridget E. Gurtler, "Synthetic

Conception: Artificial Insemination and the Transformation of Reproduction and Family in Nineteenth- and Twentieth-Century America" (PhD diss., Rutgers University, 2013), 317, 342.

3. Risa Cromer, "Making the Ethnic Embryo: Enacting Race in US Embryo Adoption," *Medical Anthropology* 38, no. 7 (2019): 603–19, esp. 608, 614. See also Daisy Deomampo, "Racialized Commodities: Race and Value in Human Egg Donation," *Medical Anthropology* 38, no. 7 (2019): 603–633, esp. 623.

4. Charlotte Kroløkke, "Click a Donor: Viking Masculinity on the Line," *Journal of Consumer Culture* 9, no. 1 (March 2009): 7–30, esp. 16; Elizabeth F. S. Roberts, "Resources and Race: Assisted Reproduction in Ecuador," *Reproductive BioMedicine and Society Online* 2 (June 2016): 47–53, esp. 51.

5. Tessa Moll, "Making a Match: Curating Race in South African Gamete Donation," *Medical Anthropology* 38, no. 7 (2019): 588–602, esp. 593; see also Deomampo, "Racialized Commodities," 625.

6. Moll, "Making a Match," 597; see also Deomampo, "Racialized Commodities," 629.

7. Amrita Pande, "'Mix or Match?': Transnational Fertility Industry and White Desirability," *Medical Anthropology* 40, no. 4 (2021): 335–347, esp. 335, 343. Emphasis in the original.

8. Lucy van de Wiel, *Freezing Fertility: Oocyte Cryopreservation and the Gender Politics of Aging* (New York: New York University Press, 2020), 192.

9. Camisha A. Russell, *The Assisted Reproduction of Race* (Bloomington: Indiana University Press, 2018), 46.

10. Rajani Bhatia, "The Development of Sex-Selective Reproductive Technologies within Fertility, Inc. and the Anticipation of Lifestyle Sex Selection," in *Selective Reproduction in the 21st Century*, ed. Ayo Wahlberg and Tine M. Gammeltoft (Cham: Palgrave Macmillan, 2017), 45–66, esp. 55, 61. The US Food and Drug Administration (FDA) has not approved MicroSort as of April 2022.

11. Christina Weis, "Changing Fertility Landscapes: Exploring the Reproductive Routes and Choices of Fertility Patients from China for Assisted Reproduction in Russia," *Asian Bioethics Review* 13 (2021): 7–22, esp. 18.

12. Gena Corea, *The Mother Machine: Reproductive Technologies from Artificial Insemination to Artificial Wombs* (New York: Harper & Row, 1985), 289.

13. Corea, *Mother Machine*, 123, 176–177.

14. Jennifer Parks, "Rethinking Radical Politics in the Context of Assisted Reproductive Technology," *Bioethics* 23, no. 1 (January 2009): 20–27, esp. 25n28.

15. Amel Alghrani, *Regulating Assisted Reproductive Technologies: New Horizons* (Cambridge: Cambridge University Press, 2018), 12.

16. Katharine Dow, *Making a Good Life: An Ethnography of Nature, Ethics, and Reproduction* (Princeton, NJ: Princeton University Press, 2016), 194. United Nations, Declaration of Human Rights, accessed April 24, 2022, https://www.un.org/en/about-us/universal-declaration-of-human-rights; González-Santos, *Portrait of Assisted Reproduction in Mexico*, 171.

17. Loretta J. Ross and Rickie Solinger, *Reproductive Justice: An Introduction* (Oakland: University of California Press, 2017), 69.

18. Ross and Solinger, *Reproductive Justice*, 9, 17 (emphases in original); Diane Tober, *Romancing the Sperm: Shifting Biopolitics and the Making of Modern Families* (New Brunswick, NJ: Rutgers University Press, 2018), 190.

19. Sebastian Mohr and Lene Koch, "Transforming Social Contracts: The Social and Cultural History of IVF in Denmark," *Reproductive BioMedicine and Society Online* 2 (June 2016): 88–96, esp. 92; Laura Mamo, *Queering Reproduction: Achieving Pregnancy in the Age of Technoscience* (Durham, NC: Duke University Press, 2007), 56; "French Parliament Votes to Extend IVF Rights to Lesbians and Single Women," *The Guardian*, June 29, 2021, https://www.theguardian.com/world/2021/jun/29/french-parliament-votes-to-extend-ivf-rights-to-lesbians-and-single-women.

20. Damien W. Riggs et al., "Men, Trans/Masculine, and Non-Binary People Negotiating Conception: Normative Resistance and Inventive Pragmatism," *International Journal of Transgender Health* 22, nos. 1–2 (2021): 6–17, esp. 15, 11.

21. Olivia J. Fischer, "Non-Binary Reproduction: Stories of Conception, Pregnancy, and Birth," *International Journal of Transgender Health*, 22, nos. 1–2 (2021): 77–88, esp. 84.

22. Judith Lasker and Susan Borg, *In Search of Parenthood* (Philadelphia: Temple University Press, 1994), 148; Robin E. Jensen, *Infertility: Tracing the History of a Transformative Term* (University Park: Pennsylvania State University Press, 2016), 159.

23. Georgina M. Chambers et al., "The Economic Impact of Assisted Reproductive Technology: A Review of Selected Developed Countries," *Fertility and Sterility* 91, no. 6 (June 2009): 2281–2294; Melissa B. Jacoby, "The Debt Financing of Parenthood," *Law and Contemporary Problems* 72, no. 3 (Summer 2009): 147–176, esp. 162.

24. Manuela Perrotta and Josie Hamper, "The Crafting of Hope: Contextualizing Add-Ons in the Treatment Trajectories of IVF Patients," *Social Science & Medicine* 287, no. 114317 (2021): 1–8, esp. 4, 6.

25. Dow, *Making a Good Life*, 97.

Chapter 6

1. Toni Weschler, *Taking Charge of Your Fertility: The Definitive Guide to Natural Birth Control, Pregnancy Achievement, and Reproductive Health*, 20th anniversary ed. (New York: HarperCollins, 2015), 257; see also Susan Martha Kahn, "The Mirth of the Clinic: Field Notes from an Israeli Fertility Center," in *Kin, Gene, Community: Reproductive Technologies among Jewish Israelis*, ed. Daphna Birenbaum-Carmeli and Yoram S. Carmeli (New York: Berghahn Books, 2010), 296–317, esp. 311.

2. Matthew Schmidt and Lisa Jean Moore, "Constructing a 'Good Catch,' Picking a Winner: The Development of Technosemen and the Deconstruction of the Monolithic Male," in *Cyborg Babies: From Techno-Sex to Techno-Tots*, ed. Robbie Davis-Floyd and Joseph Dumit (New York: Routledge, 1998), 21–39, esp. 26, 27.

3. Charlotte Kroløkke, "Click a Donor: Viking Masculinity on the Line," *Journal of Consumer Culture* 9, no. 1 (March 2009): 7–30, esp. 24; Ayo Wahlberg, *Good Quality: The Routinization of Sperm Banking in China* (Oakland: University of California Press, 2018), 140.

4. Wahlberg, *Good Quality*, 142; Li Wu et al., "Association between Ambient Particulate Matter Exposure and Semen Quality in Wuhan, China," *Environment International* 98 (January 2017): 219–228.

5. Lisa Jean Moore, *Sperm Counts: Overcome by Man's Most Precious Fluid* (New York: New York University Press, 2007), 150.

6. Weschler, *Taking Charge of Your Fertility*, 235, 274.

7. Willem Ombelet, "The Development in In-Vitro Fertilization in Africa," in *In-Vitro Fertilization: The Pioneers' History*, ed. Gabor Kovacs, Peter Brinsden, and Alan DeCherney (Cambridge: Cambridge University Press, 2018), 158–171, esp. 163, 164; Rudi Campo et al., "Office Mini-Hysteroscopy," *Human Reproduction Update* 5, no. 1 (January–February 1999): 73–81; Carlo de Angelis et al., "Office Hysteroscopy and Compliance: Mini-Hysteroscopy versus Traditional Hysteroscopy in a Randomized Trial," *Human Reproduction* 18, no. 11 (November 2003): 2441–2445.

8. Trudie Gerrits, "Assisted Reproductive Technologies in Ghana: Transnational Undertakings, Local Practices, and 'More Affordable' IVF," *Reproductive BioMedicine and Society Online* 2 (June 2016): 32–38, esp. 37.

9. Laura Mamo, *Queering Reproduction: Achieving Pregnancy in the Age of Technoscience* (Durham, NC: Duke University Press, 2007), 46–47, 136, 144.

10. Mamo, *Queering Reproduction*, 144, 160.

11. John J. Billings, *The Ovulation Method: The Achievement or Avoidance of Pregnancy by a Technique Which Is Safe, Reliable and Morally Acceptable* (Melbourne:

Advocate Press, 1980); "Natural Family Planning," United States Conference of Catholic Bishops, accessed April 24, 2022, https://www.usccb.org /topics/natural-family-planning; on ovulation predictor kits, see Jenna Caitlin Healey, "Sooner or Later: Age, Pregnancy, and the Reproductive Revolution in Late Twentieth-Century America" (PhD diss., Yale University, 2016), 249–252.

12. Katie Singer, "Cycles of Hot and Cold: Trying to Learn Fertility Awareness in North America," in *Voices of the Women's Health Movement*, vol. 1, ed. Barbara Seaman with Laura Eldridge (New York: Seven Stories Press, 2012), 174–177, esp. 176.

13. Weschler, *Taking Charge of Your Fertility*, 66–67, 10.

14. Roshonara Ali et al., "Do Fertility Tracking Applications Offer Women Useful Information about Their Fertile Window?," *Reproductive BioMedicine Online* 42, no. 1 (January 2021): 273–281, esp. 276.

15. "Daysy: Your Personal Fertility Tracker," Valley Electronics AG, accessed April 24, 2022, https://daysy.me/; Niels van de Roemer et al., "The Performance of a Fertility Tracking Device," *European Journal of Contraception & Reproductive Health Care* 26, no. 2 (2021): 111–118.

16. Kylie Baldwin, "The Biomedicalization of Reproductive Ageing: Reproductive Citizenship and the Gendering of Fertility Risk," *Health, Risk, & Society* 21, nos. 5–6 (2019): 268–283, esp. 275; Pippa Grenfell et al., "Fertility and Digital Technology: Narratives of Using Smartphone App 'Natural Cycles' While Trying to Conceive," *Sociology of Health & Illness* 41, no. 1 (2021): 116–132, esp. 124, 128.

17. "2018 Assisted Reproductive Technology Fertility Clinic Success Rates Report," Centers for Disease Control and Prevention, last modified January 12, 2021, https://www.cdc.gov/art/reports/2018/fertility-clinic.html.

18. Claude Ranoux et al., "A New In Vitro Fertilization Technique: Intravaginal Culture," *Fertility and Sterility* 49, no. 4 (April 1988): 654–657; Teru Jellerette-Nolan et al., "Real-World Experience with Intravaginal Culture Using INVOCELL: An Alternative Model for Infertility Treatment," *F&S Reports* 2, no. 1 (March 2021): 9–15; Elnur Babayev and Tarun Jain, "Intravaginal Culture Using INVOCELL: Is It a Viable Option for Infertility?," *F&S Reports* 2, no. 1 (March 2021): 7–8.

19. Ombelet, "Development in In-Vitro Fertilization in Africa," 165, 164, 168; see also Willem Ombelet et al., "The tWE Lab Simplified IVF Procedure: First Births after Freezing/Thawing," *Facts, Views, & Vision in ObGyn* 6, no. 1 (March 2014): 45–49.

20. Sarah Elizabeth Richards, "Growing Cheaper Embryos for IVF inside the Vagina," *The Atlantic*, last modified July 12, 2017, https://www.theatlantic

.com/health/archive/2017/07/growing-cheaper-embryos-for-ivf-inside-the-vagina/533205; Elkin Lucena et al., "INVO Procedure: Minimally Invasive IVF as an Alternative Treatment Option for Infertile Couples," *Scientific World Journal* (2012): article ID 571596; Sarah Ferber et al., *IVF and Assisted Reproduction: A Global History* (Singapore: Palgrave Macmillan, 2020), 253.

21. Sarah Lensen et al., "How Common Is Add-On Use and How Do Patients Decide Whether to Use Them? A National Survey of IVF Patients," *Human Reproduction* 36, no. 7 (July 2021): 1854–1861, esp. 1859, 1857.

22. "Treatment Add-Ons with Limited Evidence," Human Fertilisation and Embryology Authority, accessed April 24, 2022, https://www.hfea.gov.uk/treatments/treatment-add-ons.

23. Lensen et al., "How Common Is Add-On Use?," 1857; Mohan S. Kamath et al., "Clinical Adjuncts in In Vitro Fertilization: A Growing List," *Fertility and Sterility* 112, no. 6 (December 2019): 978–986; Sarah Lensen et al., "In-Vitro Fertilization Add-Ons for the Endometrium: It Doesn't Add Up," *Fertility and Sterility* 112, no. 6 (December 2019): 987–993, esp. 990.

24. Lucy van de Wiel, *Freezing Fertility: Oocyte Cryopreservation and the Gender Politics of Aging* (New York: New York University Press, 2020), 120, 121; "Embryoscope Time-Lapse System," Vitrolife, accessed April 24, 2022, https://www.vitrolife.com/products/time-lapse-systems/embryoscope-time-lapse-system; Lucy van de Wiel et al., "The Prevalence, Promotion, and Pricing of Three IVF Add-Ons on Fertility Clinic Websites," *Reproductive BioMedicine Online* 41, no. 5 (November 2020): 801–806, esp. 803; see also Alberto Revelli et al., "Impact of the Addition of Early Embryo Viability Assessment to Morphological Evaluation on the Accuracy of Embryo Selection on Day 3 or Day 5: A Retrospective Analysis," *Journal of Ovarian Research* 12 (2019): article 73.

25. Van de Wiel, *Freezing Fertility*, 129.

26. Catherine Waldby, *The Oocyte Economy: The Changing Meaning of Human Eggs* (Durham, NC: Duke University Press, 2019), 79 (emphasis in original).

27. Van de Wiel, *Freezing Fertility*, 137, Alina Geampana and Manuela Perrotta, "Predicting Success in the Embryology Lab: The Use of Algorithmic Technologies in Knowledge Production," *Science, Technology, & Human Values* (2021): preprint, 1–22. I am grateful to Alina Geampana for some of the insights in this section.

28. "Time-Lapse Imaging," Human Fertilisation and Embryology Authority, accessed April 24, 2022, https://www.hfea.gov.uk/treatments/treatment-add-ons/time-lapse-imaging; Sarah Armstrong et al., "Add-Ons in the Laboratory: Hopeful, but Not Always Helpful," *Fertility and Sterility* 112, no. 6 (December 2019): 994–999, esp. 994–995; Jack Wilkinson et al., "Do à la Carte Menus

Serve Infertility Patients? The Ethics and Regulation of In Vitro Fertility Add-Ons," *Fertility and Sterility* 112, no. 6 (December 2019): 973–977, esp. 976.

29. Kamath et al., "Clinical Adjuncts in In Vitro Fertilization," 984.

30. Weschler, *Taking Charge of Your Fertility*, 251; Waldby, *Oocyte Economy*, 163, 180–188.

31. Cathy Herbrand, "Silences, Omissions and Oversimplification? The UK Debate on Mitochondrial Donation," *Reproductive Biomedicine and Society Online* 14 (March 2022): 53–62, esp. 58, 56.

32. The first successful uterine transplant-IVF procedure with a deceased donor occurred in Brazil in 2017: Dani Ejzenberg et al., "Livebirth after Uterine Transplantation from a Deceased Donor in a Recipient with Uterine Infertility," *Lancet* 392, 10165 (December 22, 2018–January 4, 2019): 2697–2704; A. Del Rio et al., "Uterus Transplant Update: Innovative Fertility Solutions and the Widening Horizons of Bioengineering," *European Review for Medical and Pharmacological Sciences* 25, no. 9 (2021): 3405–3410, esp. 3405; Amel Alghrani, *Regulating Assisted Reproductive Technologies: New Horizons* (Cambridge: Cambridge University Press, 2018), 13.

33. Pernilla Dahm-Kähler et al., "Uterine Transplantation for Fertility Preservation in Patients with Gynecologic Cancer," *International Journal of Gynecological Cancer* 31, no. 3 (March 2021): 371–378; Natasha Hammond-Browning and Si Liang Yao, "Deceased Donation Uterus Transplantation: A Review," *Transplantology* 2 (no. 2, 2021): 140–148; Benjamin P. Jones et al., "Uterine Transplantation Using Living Donation: A Cross-Sectional Study Assessing Perceptions, Acceptability, and Suitability," *Transplantation Direct* 7, no. 3 (March 2021): e673; Lisa Guntram, "May I Have Your Uterus? The Contribution of Considering Complexities Preceding Live Uterus Transplantation," *Medical Humanities* 47, no. 4 (December 2021): 425–437, esp. 425, 429.

34. Alghrani, *Regulating Assisted Reproductive Technologies*, 111, 121–123, 143.

35. Alghrani, *Regulating Assisted Reproductive Technologies*, 61; Ferber et al., *IVF and Assisted Reproduction*, 247.

36. Alghrani, *Regulating Assisted Reproductive Technologies*, 228, 238–239; Felicitas Falck et al., "Undergoing Pregnancy and Childbirth as Trans Masculine in Sweden: Experiencing and Dealing with Structural Discrimination, Gender Norms, and Microaggressions in Antenatal Care, Delivery, and Gender Clinics," *International Journal of Transgender Health* 22, nos. 1–2 (2021): 42–53, esp. 43; Chloë Rogers et al., "A Retrospective Study of Positive and Negative Determinants of Gamete Storage in Transgender and Gender-Diverse Patients," *International Journal of Transgender Health* 22, nos. 1–2 (2021): 167–178, esp. 175.

37. Olivia J. Fischer, "Non-Binary Reproduction: Stories of Conception, Pregnancy, and Birth," *International Journal of Transgender Health*, 22, nos. 1–2 (2021): 77–88, esp. 80; Rogers et al., "A Retrospective Study of Positive and Negative Determinants," 167–168.

38. Ethics Committee of the American Society for Reproductive Medicine, "Access to Fertility Services by Transgender Persons: An Ethics Committee Opinion," *Fertility and Sterility* 104, no. 5 (November 2015): 1111–1115; Damien W. Riggs et al., "Men, Trans/Masculine, and Non-Binary People Negotiating Conception: Normative Resistance and Inventive Pragmatism," *International Journal of Transgender Health* 22, nos. 1–2 (2021): 6–17, esp. 15.

39. Alghrani, *Regulating Assisted Reproductive Technologies*, 258.

40. Anna Louie Sussman, "The Promise and Perils of the New Fertility Entrepreneurs," *The New Yorker*, May 19, 2021, https://www.newyorker.com/tech/annals-of-technology/the-promise-and-perils-of-the-new-fertility-entrepreneurs.

41. Van de Wiel, *Freezing Fertility*, 111, 113; Lucy van de Wiel, "The Speculative Turn in IVF: Egg Freezing and the Financialization of Fertility," *New Genetics and Society: Critical Studies of Contemporary Biosciences* 39, no. 3 (2020): 306–326.

42. Van de Wiel, *Freezing Fertility*, 118.

43. Sussman, "The Promise and Perils of the New Fertility Entrepreneurs"; Kate Clark, "Kindbody Raises $15M, Will Open a 'Fertility Bus' with Mobile Testing & Assessments," *Tech Crunch*, April 17, 2019, https://techcrunch.com/2019/04/16/kindbody-raises-15m-will-open-a-fertility-bus-with-mobile-testing-assessments.

44. Fischer, "Non-Binary Reproduction," 84.

45. Donna J. Drucker, *Contraception: A Concise History* (Cambridge, MA: MIT Press, 2020).

46. Sandra P. González-Santos, *A Portrait of Assisted Reproduction in Mexico: Scientific, Political, and Cultural Interactions* (Cham: Palgrave Macmillan, 2020), 187.

FURTHER READING

Davis, Gayle, and Tracey Loughran, eds. *The Palgrave Handbook of Infertility in History*. London: Palgrave Macmillan, 2017.

Ferber, Sarah, Nicola J. Marks, and Vera Mackie. *IVF and Assisted Reproduction: A Global History*. Singapore: Palgrave Macmillan, 2020.

Franklin, Sarah. *Embodied Progress: A Cultural Account of Assisted Conception*. London: Routledge, 1997.

Kahn, Susan Martha. *Reproducing Jews: A Cultural Account of Assisted Conception in Israel*. Durham, NC: Duke University Press, 2000.

Marsh, Margaret, and Wanda Ronner. *The Pursuit of Parenthood: Reproductive Technology from Test-Tube Babies to Uterus Implants*. Baltimore, MD: Johns Hopkins University Press, 2019.

Pfeffer, Naomi. *The Stork and the Syringe: A Political History of Reproductive Medicine*. Cambridge: Polity Press, 1993.

Swanson, Kara W. "The Birth of the Sperm Bank." *Annals of Iowa* 71 (Summer 2012): 241–276.

Thompson, Charis. *Making Parents: The Ontological Choreography of Reproductive Technologies*. Cambridge, MA: MIT Press, 2005.

van de Wiel, Lucy. *Freezing Fertility: Oocyte Cryopreservation and the Gender Politics of Aging*. New York: New York University Press, 2020.

Wahlberg, Ayo. *Good Quality: The Routinization of Sperm Banking in China*. Oakland: University of California Press, 2018.

Waldby, Catherine. *The Oocyte Economy: The Changing Meaning of Human Eggs*. Durham, NC: Duke University Press, 2019.

INDEX

Note: Page numbers in *italics* indicate illustrations.

Eggs
 artificial stimulation, 82
 freezing, 85, 90–97, 110–111,
  184
 retrieval techniques, 66, 69, 81–
  85, 123–124
 survival period, 43
 vitrification, 90–92, 94, 97
Embryo flushing, 83
Embryology, 19
Embryonic stem cells (ESC), 175
Embryos
 freezing of, 82, 90
 medium/culture for, 67–69, 85
 religious issues, 107–108
 three-parent, 175
 time-lapse imaging for selection
  of, 172–174
 treatment of, 107–108
EmbryoScope, 172
Endocrinology, 33
Endometrial scratching, 171
Endometriosis, 59, 66, 70, 117
Enslaved women, as research
  subjects, 18–19, 22
Estes, William L., Jr., 35–36
Estes, William L., Sr., 35
Estrogen, 33
Ethical/moral issues. *See also*
  Religious issues
 egg donors and surrogates, 11, 12,
  112–113
 embryo freezing, 82
 IVM and MDNA, 175–177
 overview, 8
 queer families, 181–182
 savior siblings, 105–106
 selective reproduction, 79–81,
  136–138

status of embryos, 108
 storage, disposal, and use of
  gametes and embryos, 106–108
Eugenics, 79, 151
European Society of Human
  Reproduction and Embryology
  (ESHRE), 91, 106–107

Fallopian tubes
 blocked/damaged, 7, 11, 35–37,
  40–41, 59, 61, 70, 83, 158
 surgical placement of egg and
  sperm in, 75–76
Falloscopy, 158
Family and kinship. *See also*
  Motherhood; Paternity; Queer
  families
 meanings of, affected by ARTs,
  129, 150–151, 187
 overview of issues, 9
 racial considerations, 130–136
 reproductive justice, 141–146
Family balancing, 137
Fanconi anemia, 106
Farris, Edmond J., 32
Fehling, Hermann, 27
Feminism
 critiques of ARTs, 9, 11, 138–140,
  143
 and racial considerations, 131
 United Nations Declaration of
  Human Rights, 143
 women's health movement, 160,
  163
Ferber, Sarah, 125
Fertility awareness method (FAM),
  164
Fertility extension technologies,
  93–94